There's more to medical care ...

BUILDING PATIENT/DOCTOR TRUST

Copyright @ 2005 by Frank H. Boehm, M.D.

Editorial Supervision: Julie Boehm and Debbie Bone

All rights reserved. No part of this book may be reproduced in any form without written permission from the author. Earlier versions of the essays in this book were originally published in The Nashville *TENNESSEAN*.

Design by MGroup, Nashville, Tennessee

Back Cover Photograph by Dennis Wile

ISBN: 0-9772351-0-6

Inquiries should be addressed to: Dr. Frank Boehm, 202 Burlington Place, Nashville, TN 37215

Printed in the USA

www.DoctorBoehm.com

There's more to medical care ...

BUILDING PATIENT/DOCTOR TRUST

FRANK H. BOEHM, M.D.

DEDICATION

To my colleagues who helped teach me
the complexities of medical care

To my patients who helped teach me about
the depth of feelings and emotions surrounding medical care

and to my wife Julie and my children
who never stop teaching me about love

TABLE OF CONTENTS

From the Author III

Trust 1
Patient Responsibility 5
Choosing your Doctor 9
The New Hippocratic Oath 11
Informed Consent 14
Sleep Deprivation 17
Patient Safety 20
The Uninsured ... A Time for Change 23
Medical Malpractice 27
Defensive Medicine 29
I'm Sorry 32
Bedside Manners 35
Men Cry, Too 37
Boutique Medicine 39
The Value of Nurses 41
Doctors and the Media 45
Ethics of Multiple Births 48
What to Do 50
When Life Begins 52
Abortion and Gestational Limits 54
Abortion for Gender Selection 56
Partial Birth Abortion 58
Emergency Contraception 62
Morality and the Pharmacist 65
Oregon and Physician-Assisted Suicide 68
Marijuana as Medicine 71
Free Needles 73
The Mystery and Pain of Suicide 75
Insanity or Murder: Postpartum Depression 78

It's In Your Head 81
Sexual Information 84
Heart of a Woman 86
Get Off the Couch 89
The Bible and Your Health 92
Too Many Choices 95
Can We Know Too Much 98
The Perfect Child 100
Birth Order Matters 103
When Our Children Become Adults 105
It's All About Genes 108
The *Big Chill* Weekend 110
As Old As You Feel 113
The Sorrow of Losing a Pet 115
The Good Old Days are Now 117
Life's Bookends 119
Living Too Long 122
Spirituality and Health 124
The Power of Touch 127
Holding Onto Hope 129
Healing With Words 131
Heroes in Medicine 133
Practicing Medicine 136
Doctors: Too Few or Too Many? 139
The Price of Being a Doctor 142
Nothing Has Changed: Business as Usual 144
Genetics and Pain 147
Emergency Room Medicine 149
Obesity and Health Care Costs 151
Conflict of Interest in Medicine 153
Thank You or Bribe? 156
Passage of Time 158

FROM THE AUTHOR

The patient/doctor relationship is in trouble. What was once a close and trusting relationship is now becoming distant and suspicious. That is unfortunate and quite troubling.

For doctors, a close, helpful and trusting relationship with their patients is one of the main reasons most choose to become doctors in the first place.

In most cases, it is a doctor who first touches us when we are born and it is a doctor who is often the last to touch us before we die. Between these two bookends of life, we experience a multitude of encounters with the men and women of medicine whose responsibility is to help us regain and maintain our health and well-being.

There are many reasons for this fractured relationship between doctor and patient: millions of Americans without health care insurance, overcrowded emergency rooms and doctor offices, too little time available to spend between doctor and patient, patient safety, a disparity of medical outcome for minorities, a malpractice environment which all lead to defensive medical practices, suspicious doctors and skeptical patients.

At the root of these reasons lies an important common denominator, the lack of communication between patient and doctor. There was a time when doctors went to the home to dispense care.

During those visits family members and their doctor got to know each other. They often shared a piece of cake or a cup of coffee during the visit, and over the years developed a trusting relationship. Unfortunately today, with so little time available for doctors to visit with patients, we lack the means to establish this critically important and necessary relationship.

In my first book, *Doctors Cry, Too: Essays from the Heart of a Physician,* I shared much of my personal life, as well as profound medical experiences with many of my patients, in an effort to show the heart of a physician and how doctors care very much about their patients.

In *Building Patient/Doctor Trust* I deal with the many challenges surrounding medical care and politics, such as patient responsibility, choosing a doctor, abortion, medical malpractice, and the uninsured, to name a few. And I continue in my effort to help patient and doctor better understand each challenge in the hope of regaining a close and trusting relationship.

Doctors should let their patients know more about who they are and what they believe. In return, patients have a responsibility to help their doctor take better care of them by understanding the many complexities in today's medical profession. Opening lines of communication between patient and doctor is a good place to start to accomplish this basic trusting relationship.

There is more to medical care than merely dispensing medical care. It also means sharing life's experiences and opinions between patient and doctor.

It is my hope that after reading *Building Patient/Doctor Trust* you will understand that in addition to your medical problems there are a wealth of other issues that can be discussed with your doctor to enhance communication and improve the relationship.

Doctors have many opinions concerning health care, what follows here are many of mine. ■

TRUST

Trust is the glue that binds one human to another. It is the foundation which brings each of us peace and comfort, tranquility and calm. Without trust we are shipwrecked on a sea of confusion, insecurity and fear.

Trust is not easily achieved and often takes time to be affixed to the soul, as is the case with the building of friendship or love. Yet regardless of how long it takes us to achieve a sense of trust, it is this human feeling that allows us to feel safe and protected.

In the dispensing of medical care, trust is paramount. Patients who trust their doctor to help them through the rigors of maintaining or attaining good health are rewarded by a sense of peace. Without it, patients are often confused and afraid. It is this trust between patient and physician that is critical to an effective relationship and vital to achieving positive results.

When strapping yourself into an airplane seat, that sense of trust comes automatically. You are about to be lifted 35,000 feet into the air and flown to a destination hundreds or thousands of miles away, yet, you nonetheless feel an element of trust. Obviously, part of that trust comes from the fact that you know it takes an incredible amount of training and experience to become an airline pilot.

However, a more guttural reason comes from the understanding that these unknown men and women sitting in the cockpit have a self-serving reason to assure your safety. Your well-being is tied into their well-being. If you go down, they go down. Hence, you are infused with an almost instantaneous feeling of trust.

It is this same level of trust that is so critical to the relationship between a patient and doctor. In most instances, however, that feeling of trust takes more time to develop.

Knowing that your doctor has passed the rigors of years of medical training, has been certified by a number of prestigious organizations and has had years of medical experience, is not enough to guarantee unconditional trust as occurs with an airline pilot.

Because of this, an additional layer is necessary to connect doctor and patient to create a feeling of closeness. One way this can be achieved is as simple as casual conversations during office visits. The more our patients know who their physician is as an individual, the more our patients will feel a sense of caring and trust.

I have often marveled at the fact that many of my patients, once feeling this sense of trust, will allow me to make critical decisions for them in times of their greatest need. I am honored by this trust, yet I know that it did not happen just because I wore a white coat, carried a stethoscope and was called "Doctor."

While I did have all the trappings of a physician, my patients began to feel a sense of trust in my care because they also began to know who I was and what were some of my fundamental thoughts and beliefs.

The more each knows about the other, the better the physician is in taking care of his or her patient and the more the patient feels trust in the physician. In an ever-increasing medical technological environment in which human touch is easily replaced by machines and drugs, it is imperative for doctors to achieve and maintain a patient's trust through expert care dosed along the way with personal interactions.

A 2002 survey revealed that while Americans have great faith in each other, they have lost considerable faith in certain professionals, such as CEOs, stockbrokers, Catholic priests and HMO administrators. The question is, are doctors next?

While society in general still trusts and respects doctors, we may soon find our profession suffering a fate similar to that of other professions. In some ways, we are already beginning to witness erosion of trust in medical care.

Consider the following: two Institute of Medicine reports, one claiming that there were as many as 98,000 accidental hospital deaths each year, and a report critical of the disparity of medical care and outcome experienced by minorities in this country; sporadic reports of doctors performing unnecessary operations or operating on the wrong part of the body; reports of radiologists missing breast cancers when reading mammograms; doctors implanting organs from donors with the wrong blood type to critically ill recipients; an incident in Boston where a surgeon actually left the operating room during surgery to make a bank deposit.

There is also a growing concern of conflict of interest by physicians as they attempt to maintain a workable bottom line in an era of managed care medicine.

It has been reported that nine out of ten medical experts who participate in writing national guidelines for treating numerous diseases and conditions have financial ties to the pharmaceutical companies that manufacture the drugs included in the guidelines, and that these financial ties are almost never disclosed.

In addition, recent studies have revealed hormone replacement for post menopausal women was associated with an increased risk of heart attacks, thereby totally changing recommendations made by doctors on how to treat menopause; studies revealing an increased death rate in patients using the highly recommended arthritis medications; and the newly released warnings that medication used to treat adolescent depression could lead to suicide.

Is there any wonder that Americans are beginning to ask the question, "Who can we trust?"

Patients yearn for a caring, and trusting relationship with their physicians. To build trust in today's environment, doctors need to not only administer professional care but also show patients they care about them by revealing their personal, emotional and humanistic side.

There are many ways this can be achieved. In addition to adding casual conversation, doctors should share personal life experiences or take the time to discuss an important issue of the day during office visits.

Physicians can also show patients they care by sitting on the side of hospital beds, holding a hand or putting their arm around a patient, writing condolence letters to a patient's family, attending a patient's funeral or personally calling patients with important medical test results.

Physicians need to state what is known or not known to be medically proven by evidence-based medicine when discussing diagnosis and treatment and to make sure their patients understand the difference.

Because we do not have all the answers, it is our responsibility to assure that our patients are fully informed on the risk-benefit aspects of medical treatment plans. We must also provide a foundation of absolute confidentiality and truth telling as we dispense care to our patients. It is vital that we be our patients' most ardent advocate.

Patients care very much how their doctor feels about what happens to them, and these feelings can significantly influence general attitudes about the medical profession. By learning more about us and witnessing our personal, emotional and humanistic side, patients can develop the trust that is paramount to the practice of quality medicine.

If physicians are to avoid the loss of trust that so many other professionals have encountered, we must pay attention to these simple measures. It is possible, in this confusing and frustrating era of medical practice and malpractice claims to show patients that we care and that we can be trusted.

In a world where the house-calling physician no longer exists, it is vital for doctors to strive to regain and maintain trust in the medical profession.

• • •

PATIENT RESPONSIBILITY

For most of us, it is a physician who first touches us when we are born and it is a physician who is often the last to touch us before we die. Between these two boundaries of life, we experience a multitude of encounters with the men and women of medicine who help us regain, as well as, maintain our health and well-being.

It would seem, therefore, that each of us has a unique opportunity to establish one of life's special relationships, one between patient and physician.

Patients yearn for a close, caring, and compassionate relationship with their doctor, unfortunately, for a variety of reasons, many Americans are not able to develop this special relationship.

The absence of health care insurance is one obstacle to a patient developing a nurturing, long-term relationship with a physician. But often, even those who are fortunate to have a personal physician do not achieve an ideal relationship.

While there has been much attention given to what physicians should do to achieve a positive relationship with their patients, little has been said about a patient's responsibility. I believe patients also have a responsibility for making sure they receive the care they expect and desire from their doctors.

I am amazed that many people often spend more time picking out a car or television set than they do in choosing a doctor. During the past few years, in my travels around the country to promote my first book, *Doctors Cry, Too*, I have heard an often re-occurring comment: "My doctor always seems so rushed and doesn't appear to take an interest in me or my health concerns."

Because this problem does exist for many patients, I have come up with several guidelines for patients to consider as they go about finding a physician who will meet their needs:

- Learn as much as you can about your medical condition. Go to libraries, the Internet, or ask your doctor for articles that will help you understand many of the complicated issues surrounding your health. A well-informed patient is easier to care for.

- Before arriving at your doctor's appointment, write down questions you want answered, or issues you want to discuss related to diagnosis, treatment, side effects, or prognosis. During the hectic pace of a doctor's visit, you can easily forget what you wanted to discuss or the questions you need answered. Remember that there are no stupid questions.

- If possible, take a close relative or friend with you. When hearing medical information and especially distressing or bad news, many patients do not hear what doctors tell them. Having another, less nervous, pair of ears may prove helpful on the ride home. If this is not possible, taking notes may be helpful. If you didn't understand something, don't be afraid to ask your doctor to repeat what was said.

- Patients are more comfortable, attentive and thorough when discussing their medical complaints while fully clothed. Ask your doctor to talk to you before you get undressed for the examination. For that same reason, it is best to redress before once again discussing your medical condition and course of action.

- Don't always feel your doctor has the best answer for you. Be prepared to ask about alternative treatments that may be available. A good physician will be glad to explain the risks and benefits of any reasonable alternative treatment plan.

- If you aren't comfortable with your doctor's opinion, ask for a second opinion. If your doctor has a problem with this, consider finding a new doctor. Good physicians are glad to supply patients with names of competent physicians who you can visit for a second opinion. A second opinion that concurs with your doctor's diagnosis can help build trust and confidence thus reducing the need for other such opinions in the future. A second opinion can also prevent treatment for a wrong diagnosis.

- Once you begin treatment, let your doctor know of any problems that develop. It is also a good idea to call your doctor's office when you are improving and your treatment is going well. Like everyone else, doctors enjoy hearing good news.

- Be aware of *patient autonomy*. This means you have the right to deny a particular course of action and say no to your doctor's treatment plan, or even suggest another form of treatment. Your doctor should explain the risks and benefits of a course of action versus any treatment you suggest. Just be sure you fully understand the risks involved in whatever decision you make.

- If you feel rushed or do not feel your doctor has answered your questions, speak up! A simple "Doctor, can you please sit down and go over this again, I don't understand (or I am feeling rushed)" works quite well.

- If your insurance company is not cooperating, ask your doctor or the business office if there is something you can do to help resolve the issue. Health care should be a team effort, and you and your doctor are on the same team.

If after you try these suggestions your physician still does not fulfill your health care needs, perhaps it is time to find another doctor. Just as patients depend on their physician, physicians also depend on their patients. Patient responsibility is an important factor in maintaining good health.

From birth to death and all that comes between, doctors and patients should work together in a spirit of cooperation and support. Only in this way can the relationship between physician and patient be a fulfilling, positive experience. Considering what is at stake, it is too important to settle for less.

. . .

CHOOSING YOUR DOCTOR

While there are numerous items on the subject of health care, one of the most emotional is that of having to change doctors. Surveys agree that Americans are the most upset about changes in health care plans when they are forced to find another doctor. Can you blame them?

The entire process of finding the right doctor best suited for you and your health problems is multifactorial, difficult and often quite frustrating. However, when that right physician is finally found, a sense of peace is established.

One aspect in finding the right physician not often thought about, concerns the perception that all doctors are basically alike. After all, one car mechanic fixes a car pretty much as another one does, so perhaps one doctor will do what is needed just as any other doctor. WRONG!

While a car can be reduced to a subtotal of workable parts, the human body and spirit is an incredibly complicated, intricate living organism with interwoven layer upon layer of physical, emotional, psychological, spiritual and societal needs — hardly a comparable scenario.

Primary to understanding that physicians are not all alike is the fact that the approximately 700,000 American physicians are, except for basic similarities such as a love of science and a sincere desire to provide for the sick, as different as the individuals who live in your neighborhood.

Those of us who train young men and women to become physicians are quite adept at witnessing these vast differences in communication skills, personalities, mannerisms and interests.

As individuals, physicians are as different as snowflakes. Some are adept at revealing compassion and concern, while others are not. Some are able to choose more easily and readily the proper words to teach, inform and explain what may be happening, what is happening and what is about to happen. Some physicians have an inherent ability to exude body language that is positive, warm and comforting while others struggle to convey these feelings.

In our differences, however, we are much alike. Residing in most physicians is concern and compassion for a patient's well-being that is often not appreciated by patients. Residing in most physicians is a sincere and honest feeling of wanting to help, be liked, appreciated and feel needed.

An insurance company or medical care plan can no more help you choose the right physician than a computer can find the right person for you to marry.

Only after trial and error can you decide when you have found the physician who understands your needs, who is able to explain to you what is needed in ways that you can best understand, and who can bring you comfort and peace as you go through life's inevitable ups and downs, and most importantly, one whom you can trust.

The quest, therefore, to find that perfect doctor is often difficult, time-consuming and frustrating. Since each patient is as complicated as each doctor, the discovery of the right physician can be a lucky and rewarding event.

Currently many health care plans offer limited lists of physicians from which a patient may choose. I suggest, to any politician who may be toying with the idea of changing our health care landscape, that whatever you do, do not mess with a patient's right to choose their own physician.

While our plans are now based on achieving an improved economic bottom line, I still believe that Americans should not be forced to leave physician's they have grown to trust, admire and with whom they feel comfortable.

• • •

THE NEW HIPPOCRATIC OATH

Approximately 2500 years ago Hippocrates wrote his famous oath for physicians to take before embarking on a medical career. It outlined a number of rules that physicians must follow to comply with a code of conduct in the dispensing of medical care to patients.

The original oath required physicians to swear to do all that is possible to cure the sick; to keep patients from harm and injustice; to not give a deadly drug to anyone if asked for it; to not give to a woman an abortive remedy nor to perform surgery on any patient; to visit the sick only for their benefit remaining free of all intentional injustice, mischief and sexual relations; and to maintain strict confidentiality on all matters relating to patients.

That same oath, though modified over the years, is still taken today by many of the graduating medical students in the 125 medical schools in America.

However, much has changed in the medical profession over the past 2500 years, so I was not surprised to read that a group of doctors in the United States and Europe had published a new medical oath that many believe will replace the ancient, outdated Hippocratic oath.

That new oath is called "A Physician Charter." This new charter was written in an attempt to address current issues surrounding the practice of medicine, most of which did not exist in ancient days.

One of the issues addressed is the concern "about what is an increasing mercantile environment" says one of the authors of the Charter. Today's medical profession is under enormous pressures to not only cure the sick but also maintain a workable bottom line.

Doctors are making less money despite taking more patients into their practices, and at the same time are being pressured to adopt a cost benefit mentality in dispensing their care. Consequently, many doctors are being tempted by pharmaceutical and medical device companies to accept gifts, free trips, and even cash to sell more drugs and products. The Charter authors hope that this new pledge will encourage physicians to avoid falling prey to this current climate in modern medicine.

The issue of conflict of interest has also become a real concern for the medical profession. The Physician Charter addresses this important issue of avoiding physician conflict of interest.

Conditions which exist in the medical profession today are tempting doctors to modify their commitment to patient welfare. Art Caplan, nationally recognized medical ethicist at the University of Pennsylvania was quoted in the *New York Times* as saying "Today, the practice is pulled every day to be more of a business. That is the wrong ethic."

Dr. Caplan and others in the medical field hope that this new oath will be widely disseminated throughout the medical profession and adopted as the new oath to be taken at graduation and followed throughout a practitioner's life.

The Physician Charter contains three fundamental principles and ten professional responsibilities. The three principles include the principles of patient welfare, autonomy, and social justice.

The principle of patient welfare is based on "a dedication to serving the interest of the patient and contributes to the trust that is central to the physician-patient relationship. Market forces, societal pressures, and administrative exigencies must not compromise this principle."

The principle of autonomy stresses the absolute responsibility to "be honest with patients and empower them to make informed decisions about their treatment." The Charter further states that "patient's decisions about their care must be paramount, as long as those decisions are in keeping with ethical practice and do not lead to demands for inappropriate care."

The principle of social justice includes the fair distribution of health care resources. The Charter is quite emphatic on this point. "Physicians should work actively to eliminate discrimination in health care, whether based on race, gender, socioeconomic status, ethnicity, religion, or any other social category."

The ten responsibilities in the Charter are listed as physician commitments and include the commitment to: professional competence, honesty, patient confidentiality, maintaining appropriate relations with patients, improving quality of care, improving access to care, a just distribution of finite resources, scientific knowledge, maintaining trust by managing conflicts of interest, and finally, to professional responsibilities.

There was a time when wearing a white coat and a stethoscope was enough to engender trust. Those days no longer exist because times have changed and Americans are not sure whom they can trust.

It is paramount for the medical profession to rededicate itself to the principles and commitments spelled out in The Physician Charter.

• • •

INFORMED CONSENT

A good friend called me in utter frustration. "Why can't the medical profession accept the fact that high technology is not the total answer to every medical problem?" she asked with a notable high pitch in her voice.

Having just undergone a new technique which destroys the lining of the uterus, and eliminated the need to have a hysterectomy, she was now having considerable postoperative problems and was very concerned as well as frustrated.

According to her, she was told that this "simple procedure" would be performed as an outpatient and she would be able to return to work in just a few days. After having to stay in the hospital for three days, being readmitted days later, requiring blood transfusions and then having considerable side effects for three weeks, my friend was very upset.

I attempted to comfort her, but I knew it would not be easy. She was obviously upset about the complications that occurred following what she perceived to be a simple procedure. Yet there seemed to be more as I listened to her complain about the medical profession.

It was then I asked a simple question, "Didn't your doctor explain to you that these complications might occur?"

The silence that followed this seemingly innocent question was the answer itself. "He did," she finally exclaimed, "but he said that these problems were rare and that most of his patients did well without any problems."

My friend chose to believe that everything would go as planned and that no complications would occur. The fact was, as I learned later, she had not really heard much of the discussion about complications and was only now remembering that aspect of the preoperative discussion that she had with her physician.

None of this surprised me. Over the years of explaining medical matters to patients, I have learned that many hear only a portion of what I tell them, and often it is only what they wanted to hear. A thorough medical explanation of all risks and benefits of a procedure or treatment course is called informed consent.

The question I have always asked is whether or not there truly is such a thing as informed consent?

In 1992, the Committee on Ethics of the American College of Obstetricians and Gynecologists published an eight page statement on ethical dimensions of informed consent. The Committee stated that informed consent is an ethical concept that has become intrical to contemporary medical ethics and medical practice, and that informed consent for medical treatment is an ethical requirement for medical treatment and for participation in medical research.

This statement highlights that informed consent is an expression of respect for the patient as a person and that it ensures the protection of the patient against unwanted medical treatment, while making it possible for active involvement of the patient in her or his medical planning and care.

Elements of informed consent should include: the nature of the patient's condition; the proposed treatment and the operative site; the benefits and risks of the proposed procedure, stating it is not possible to guarantee results and stating frequently occurring and significant risks; treatment alternatives, including no treatment; the consequences of no treatment and the patient should be given the opportunity to ask questions and receive additional information as requested.

I believe my friend would have been less upset with her doctor and the medical profession had she asked more questions and spent more time with her doctor during the signing of the consent form.

My friend should have made herself more knowledgeable about the procedure, either before or after the appointment with her doctor, by going to the library or using the internet to obtain more information.

She should have then written her questions down and presented them to her doctor. In addition, she probably should have brought a relative or friend to the doctor's office so as to have someone who can listen more attentively to what is discussed and then to be able to offer feedback.

My friend should have considered taking notes of what was spoken about, asked for literature on the procedure, discussed alternatives, and even requested her physician to provide her with information on how many procedures he had performed as well as how many complications he has noted in his performance of the proposed surgical treatment.

Her doctor, in turn, probably should have known his patient better. A few questions would have revealed that, in general, she was skeptical of the medical profession and more interested in a holistic approach to illness. He then could have made more attempts to make sure that she understood what was being said.

Informed consent forms are often signed too quickly and without significant deliberations. Sometimes that has to be the case in emergencies when rapid actions often precludes being able to ask all the questions or give serious thought to what is about to happen. However, when treatment does not involve an emergency decision, patients should listen carefully, ask questions, and make judgments based on all the information.

Unfortunately, most of the time, both the patient and the physician only pay lip service to the informed consent process. What often happens after that is just what happened to my friend, a very dissatisfied customer.

• • •

SLEEP DEPRIVATION

The knocking at the door was loud and persistent, as was the calling of my name. Through the fog of early sleep, both noises worked their way into a dream I had begun only minutes earlier. Finally, I awoke and sat up on the narrow cot in the on-call room at the hospital, my heart pounding and my ears ringing.

As I rose to open the door, I noticed the telephone receiver off its hook and under my pillow, and wondered how it got there. Outside my room stood a hospital security officer who had been sent to wake and summon me to the emergency room. He informed me that repeated phone calls to my room had yielded only busy signals.

Hours later, having stabilized a pregnant patient who had been involved in a car accident and preparing her for surgery, I returned to my on-call quarters, and attempted to piece the puzzle together.

Only half awakened, I had answered my phone, talked to the emergency room nurse, put the receiver under my pillow and fell back into a deep sleep, oblivious to our conversation. I had been on-call and awake for 48 hours and my mind and body were thoroughly exhausted.

Sleep deprivation is not uncommon in many professions. However, in medicine it comes as a rude awakening to young, recently graduated physicians entering the years of internship and residency training. Only the young can handle this rigorous type of on-call work.

My residency began in 1965, and for the next five years I worked every-other-night, rarely sleeping, and continuing through the following day before finally going home around 6:00 pm for a night off. We worked every-other weekend at that same pace as well, from Saturday morning until Monday evening.

On the weekends I was not on-call, I worked from Thursday morning until I was replaced Saturday morning. It was during one of these long stretches that my phone-under-the-pillow event took place. There were other such events that made me realize the on-call system in medicine needed changing.

At rounds one morning with residents, nurses and professors present, we discussed a patient who had been given a change in medication during the middle of the night. As the nurse explained to the attending physicians present, this new treatment had dramatically improved the patient's recurrent problem of restlessness and agitation during the evening hours. It was explained by the nurse that I had ordered this innovative approach.

All heads turned to me for an explanation of why I had chosen this particular therapy. Having been on-call with only an hour of sleep in the middle of the night, I could not recall ordering any such medication. Rattled, I quickly scanned the patient's chart, opened to the page of orders, and was able to regain some semblance of composure and answered the question.

Despite being congratulated by my teachers after rounds, I felt vulnerable and uneasy. If in a near sleep state I could order medication and not remember doing so later, might I do something similar on another sleepless interval of my training, but perhaps next time with a less than optimal outcome?

Night nurses will tell you that they often have to call several times to awaken young physicians on-call, then double check to be sure they are alert and understands the problem at hand. Physician fatigue also has a serious effect on a physician's attitude toward patients. A tired doctor is less able to be sympathetic, tolerant, understanding or caring.

I vividly remember one such uncaring moment early one morning during my internship in surgery. Holding an abdominal wound retractor so as to allow the surgeon to do his work in a patient's abdomen, I was trying to stay awake. The patient had been shot; his aorta severed and it was clear to all of us in the operating room that he was close to death and had little chance of survival.

It was during the second hour of surgery that I began thinking that if our patient held on and did not die for another two hours, I would not be able to get any sleep before starting another full day of work. In my state of extreme fatigue, I was actually thinking that if our patient would die, I could sleep!

Much later, reflecting on my thoughts and feelings that early morning, I was horrified. Sleeplessness can give rise to thoughts and impulses that are frighteningly inconsistent to one's normal behavior and values.

Interns and residents today are no longer subject to the on-call hours I had to endure during my training. New rules and regulations for on-call work are in place throughout the graduate medical education system, thanks in large part to one notorious case.

In 1984, Libby Zion, an 18-year-old woman, died a few hours after she had been admitted through the emergency room of a New York City hospital. Many believed her death was due in part to improper care by overworked resident physicians, and the case prompted a series of investigations which resulted in many significant changes in on-call hours. New York became the only state that had a law which limited the number of hours a doctor in training could work each week.

The Accreditation Council for Graduate Medical Education issued national guidelines that took effect in 2003, limiting the 100,000 residents in training to an average of 80 hours of work per week and limiting shifts to 24 hours followed by a 10 hour break. In addition, doctors in training must not be on-call more often than every third night and should have at least one 24 hour day each week free of patient care duties.

Studies have shown that fatigue among clinicians effect safety of patients. One study noted that performance after sleep deprivation on a task involving tracking was equivalent to performance with an unsafe blood alcohol level of 0.10 percent.

With an increasingly sick population of patients in hospitals and an increasing complexity in patient care, it is clear that the ACGME acted in response to a need for change.

While some worry that these new limitations in hours at work will compromise physician training and be overly costly to hospitals which have in the past relied heavily on residents as a source of inexpensive labor, I believe these new guidelines are good for physician education as well as for patients.

• • •

PATIENT SAFETY

America's health care system is in crisis. From large numbers of uninsured citizens, to spiraling health care costs, problems are everywhere.

Doctors are burdened with malpractice insurance premiums that in many cases are forcing them to retire or leave their practices, and hospitals cannot find enough nurses to keep beds and units open, much less provide adequate care to patients.

Added to these problems is a real concern about patient safety. That is why patient safety has become a national priority.

In the late 1990s, responding to a series of highly publicized errors, the American Medical Association along with other physician organizations and hospitals joined consumer groups to form the National Patient Safety Foundation, which performs research, educates and lobbies Congress on issues related to patient safety.

A 2000 Presidential directive required all federal departments, which provide health care to implement safety programs. As a result, in the past few years Congress appropriated over $100 million for research on patient safety. The reason for all this concern stems from collected data on patient outcomes.

Several years ago, the Institute of Medicine estimated that somewhere between 44,000 and 98,000 patients died each year from errors committed during hospitalization. This is more than the number of Americans who die each year in automobile accidents!

In addition, some experts are also claiming that there are as many as 2 million patients who suffer from hospital induced illnesses each year.

There is also the issue of medical injuries that are caused by errors of omission, such as the failure to order or perform a pap smear, mammogram, colonoscopy, or control cholesterol levels and high blood pressure.

While many of these errors of omission are not solely related to physician care, they nonetheless are problematic for a health care system that prides itself in expert care.

There have been some groups in the profession of medicine that have worked to reduce error rates. By implementing new monitoring techniques such as pulse oximeters, which monitor oxygen levels during surgery, as well as the use of critical incident analysis, standardization checklists and changes in training and supervision, mortality related to anesthesia has been significantly reduced.

Despite some improvement in reducing patient errors, however, there have been some discouraging findings. A survey conducted by the Harvard School of Public Health reported that of 831 physicians surveyed, 35% said that they or members of their family had experienced a medical error that had created a serious medical complication such as death, severe pain or long-term disability.

Thirty percent of these physicians also reported that they had witnessed a medical error that led to serious harm of patients other than their family members during the past year.

What was even more troubling, however, was that these same physicians did not seem to understand how the problem of medical errors could be addressed. Less than 25% of doctors believed that it would be effective to use computers to order drugs.

To the contrary, by implementing a computerized electronic pharmaceutical order entry system, Vanderbilt Hospital was able to reduce the medication error rate to .02% (out of 4 million doses of medication dispensed annually), and for its efforts, won a "best practices award" from the American Society of Health System Pharmacists.

The Vanderbilt electronic ordering system helps correct what Dr. Erol Amon reported in the Obstetrical and Gynecological Survey as the 5 W's; wrong drug, wrong dose, wrong patient, wrong time and wrong route.

The Harvard survey also found that few doctors were enthusiastic about using only specially trained doctors in Intensive Care Units or limiting very high risk procedures to hospitals that perform a large number of the procedures, despite considerable evidence that this approach is helpful in improving patient outcomes.

In addition, only a third of doctors surveyed felt that reducing work hours for doctors in training would be effective in reducing errors.

The survey clearly indicates that the medical profession has a long way to go in significantly reducing the number of medical errors committed each year in this country. We will have to continue educating physicians about the value of changing the system of practicing medicine that most of us have grown accustomed to.

Reform in medical practices can only be successful if doctors join in support of the changes that so many experts tell us will work to reduce medical errors.

Hopefully, with all of the problems facing the medical profession, changes will occur in the next few years, such as: a major restructuring of our reimbursement process (hopefully a single payer system), malpractice tort reform (hopefully caps on non-economic losses), a major thrust in improvements of the nursing profession (hopefully better reimbursement and improved work environment) and a pervasive change in attitude by the 700,000 doctors in America to take the problem of medical errors seriously and work to make patient safety one of our most important responsibilities.

• • •

THE UNINSURED ...
A TIME FOR CHANGE

Abba Eban once said, "History teaches us that men and nations behave wisely once they have exhausted all other alternatives." I think the United States has now exhausted all possible alternatives for providing affordable, comprehensive and universal health care insurance for Americans and, therefore, it is time for our nation to act wisely and structure a national health insurance program that ensures health care for each and every American.

Health care should not be looked upon as a privilege. I believe health care is a basic right for each and every American. Until recently it has been virtually impossible for doctors to agree on the need for a universal health care program.

Surveys now, however, indicate that after years of frustration and failure with managed care that was adopted after President Clinton's health care plan failed, a majority of doctors all across America agree that it is time for a radical change.

The prestigious Institute of Medicine announced in 2004 that it was now calling for universal health insurance in the United States. The IOM did not favor a specific plan, but did issue a checklist of five principles. The checklist stated that universal health care coverage should be 1) universal 2) continuous 3) affordable 4) sustainable and 5) should promote access to high-quality health care.

With 45 million Americans having no health care insurance, another large portion of Americans being under insured, and an even larger segment of our population being totally unsatisfied with the current way medical care is being dispensed, the average American also supports a national health insurance program.

While the wheels of progress turn slowly, it does seem that there is movement towards universal health care insurance. In an article published in the *Journal of the American Medical Association*, 8000 physicians called for single-payer, universal and comprehensive national health insurance.

Claiming that health maintenance organizations have raised medical costs by billions and infuriated doctors and patients alike, the Physicians' Group for Single-Payer National Health Insurance went on record in their support for a radical change in the way medical care is dispensed in this country.

The group listed several principles that shape their vision, the most important that "Access to comprehensive health care is a human right and it is the responsibility of a society, through its government, to ensure this right."

To achieve their vision, the Group proposes an expanded and improved version of Medicare that would cover every American for all necessary medical care. Such a program is estimated to save approximately $200 billion annually by significantly reducing administrative and other overhead costs.

Administrative costs for medical care in the United States accounts for approximately 11% of health care expenditures while the Medicare program has overhead costs of only 3%. Savings of administrative and overhead costs could allow for coverage of all uninsured Americans.

Additional funds to pay for such a program could be raised by earmarking income taxes, payroll taxes, or requiring employer contributions (keep in mind that individuals, families, and corporations would no longer have to make premium insurance payments or be burdened with out-of-pocket medical costs).

The Group stated that, "The total cost of the National Health Insurance program would be no greater (and eventually less) than those of the current fragmented system." Only a public national health care program can control a medical care process this large and complicated to realize the savings necessary to make universal health care coverage affordable. Our current system, obviously, cannot do it.

A single-payer Medicare model would have numerous benefits for patients and physicians. Ask any senior citizen what they think about Medicare and you will get a favorable response.

Patients can choose their physician, receive care without multiple obstacles imposed by the government and can obtain comprehensive health care along with some prescription benefits. The proposed National Health Insurance plan would pay for all necessary prescription medications and medical supplies, based on a national formulary, a benefit not currently available to senior citizens.

Under this new proposal, doctors could choose to be paid on a fee for service basis or be salaried and would also be freed from the burdens and expense of paperwork brought about by having to deal with numerous insurance plans, all of which have different rules to follow.

And while payment to doctors from Medicare has been reduced over the past few years, a universal plan would allow for a resetting of payment schedules for services rendered. With all Americans being able to pay for medical care, doctors and hospitals could make up for some of the reduced rates set by a universal government plan.

Almost 60 years ago, President Harry S. Truman proposed a national health care insurance plan for all Americans but failed to convince legislators and citizens that his plan should be passed.

Some 30 years ago, President Richard Nixon proposed, but failed to pass, his Comprehensive Health Insurance Program. And, in his first term in office, President Bill Clinton failed to pass his Health Security Plan for universal insurance.

With many serious problems facing medical care in this country today, it is time for our politicians to take a good look at the proposal made by the Physicians' Group for Single-Payer National Health Insurance. While this proposal is not perfect and has flaws that would need to be addressed, it is time for our government and society to begin a dialog on how to insure universal health care.

Abba Eban was right. Now that we have exhausted all other possibilities, it is time for America to act wisely and compassionately by embracing a National Health Insurance program. This proposal is a good place to start.

I am not sure what the final solution to this dilemma will be, but I am certain that we cannot continue the course we are now on. By having so many Americans uninsured and under-insured, our present system violates the basic medical ethics principle of justice, which demands fair and equal distribution of health care resources. The rising cost of medical care is also putting care out of reach for many Americans.

Health care in America is unethical, too expensive and much too frustrating for all concerned. Even our medical outcome studies reveal that we lag behind in outcome statistics. Compared to 13 comparable industrial countries America ranks 12th for over a dozen health care indicators. Japan is first, Sweden second and yes, Canada is third!

It is time for action. It is time for change.

• • •

MEDICAL MALPRACTICE

The facts speak for themselves. 80% of Obstetrician/Gynecologists in this country have been sued at least once for a claim of medical malpractice, while 25% have been sued at least four times.

Medical malpractice claims against obstetricians, as well as against physicians in various other specialties, have reached epidemic proportions. Surely there cannot be this much medical incompetence in America.

The tremendous number of medical malpractice cases filed against physicians has had a significant effect on the practice of medicine throughout this country. Faced with insurance premium fees that are rising each year, many physicians are retiring early, moving their practices to areas where malpractice insurance fees are lower or closing their offices altogether.

Physicians are increasingly attempting to avoid potential malpractice cases by over-testing and over-treating. An American Medical Association Commission Gallup poll of 1,003 doctors found that over 80% of practicing physicians order extra tests in an attempt to protect themselves against lawsuits.

This defensive type of medicine has been estimated to add over $50 billion to the annual cost of health care. The public has a right to be concerned about the effect of medical malpractice claims since it affects not only availability of care, but also the cost of medical care.

While there has been much discussion and concern on how medical malpractice claims affects the general public, there has been little discussion or concern on how these claims effect physicians.

Understanding the emotional impact of a lawsuit filed against a physician may help the public understand why doctors respond to this crisis in ways that effect the care and cost of medicine.

Obviously, some doctors practice substandard care leading to serious problems and patients should have legal recourse when this happens. However, there are many physicians being sued for bad outcomes that are not a result of negligent care.

My own experience serving as an expert to review medical malpractice claims over the past 20 years, as well as data reported in the medical literature, indicates that approximately 80% of malpractice claims lack credible evidence of substandard care with a direct link to causation (criteria used to define medical negligence).

Being sued for malpractice has been compared to Kubler-Ross's stages of death and dying. First comes denial: "This couldn't be happening to me. I'm a good doctor. I take good care of my patients." Then comes anger: "How dare they do this to me! Don't they know how hard I work and how hard I try to do the right thing?"

Bargaining comes next: "If I take very good care of my patients from now on, or if I'm real nice to the attorneys or my former patient, this lawsuit will go away."

Depression follows bargaining: "This is terrible, my career is ruined! Maybe I really did something wrong. I feel terrible." This is the stage that often negatively affects self-esteem and self-confidence as well as contributes to family conflict, substance abuse, suicide and, on occasion, a physician will decide to get out of medicine altogether.

With help and support, physicians can get to the final two stages of acceptance and hope: "I am a good doctor. Maybe I will win the case."

While medical malpractice does exist in America, our current system of addressing patient's grievances toward the outcome of their care is, in many ways, flawed and needs reform. Filing a lawsuit against a doctor affects both the cost and access of medical care.

Equally important, however, is the effect on a physician's perception of integrity, competence and professionalism. People need to know about that as well.

• • •

DEFENSIVE MEDICINE

The phrase "defensive medicine" is relatively new to the practice of medicine. When I began my practice in the early 1970s, I never heard these words being spoken, yet only a few decades later, they were on the lips of almost all my colleagues. But what do these words mean?

Defensive medicine has been defined in the medical literature as "A deviation from sound medical practice that is induced primarily by a threat of liability." In practice, defensive medicine is the ordering by doctors of supplemental care such as additional testing or treatments, avoiding risky procedures, referral to specialists for care or the refusal to take care of certain patients.

Defensive medicine is considered by many as costly, as well as unnecessary for proper medical care of patients, while adding a dimension of mistrust between doctor and patient. The practice of defensive medicine has been used as an argument for medical malpractice tort reform.

A 2005 study reported in the *Journal of the American Medical Association* noted that of a survey of 824 Pennsylvania doctors, 93% stated that they sometimes or often practiced defensive medicine because of a fear of being accused of medical malpractice. Clearly, this is a troublesome finding.

While Pennsylvania is a state with a very high rate of malpractice problems, the practice of defensive medicine is considerable even in other states. It appears that a large percentage of physicians in this country are engaging in what they consider unsound practices that exposes patients and the insurers of health care to unnecessary costs, as well as patients to potential harm.

Taken to the extreme, it is also a form of defensive medicine when young doctors in training decide not to go into a specialty of medicine because it is considered at a higher risk for malpractice claims; even though that is the specialty they most desire to practice.

Or to refuse to care for patients who have complicated problems and therefore are at a somewhat higher risk for adverse outcomes, would truly represent the practice of defensive medicine.

However, defensive medicine could be looked at as a positive rather than negative medical practice because oftentimes it may actually be beneficial to patients.

Doctors have a duty to consider most, if not all, possibilities that may be responsible for patient's symptoms, findings or complaints, which may mean ordering tests that could be considered by some as unnecessary and defensive. If, however, an unnecessary test yields a positive finding, the patient may benefit.

I am aware of many breast biopsies that were considered benign by doctors, but turned out to be malignant when an "unnecessary biopsy" was performed. I also know of instances where a symptom that appeared to be indigestion actually turned out to be a heart attack, and would not have been diagnosed had the patient not been admitted to an emergency room for a few "unnecessary tests."

Sending patients to other doctors for special care or just for a second opinion may sound like defensive medicine to some, but to me simply represents good medical judgment.

The very same kind of defensive medicine that the recently surveyed Pennsylvania doctors claimed to have practiced, could be considered comprehensive, thorough and caring. That is why I am bothered so much by the term defensive medicine.

The real medical malpractice problems confronting doctors today do not reside in the practice of defensive medicine. It resides primarily in analyzing and reducing medical errors, enhancing practices that assure patient safety, improving communication and trust between doctor and patient, and promoting team training as a model for health care systems.

Defensive medicine should perhaps be a term applied more to patients than physicians. Patients who refuse to live a healthy lifestyle need to consider practicing defensive medicine by wearing seat belts, stopping smoking, reducing the amount of fried food in their diet, taking some time each week to exercise, beginning prenatal care early in pregnancy, reducing alcohol intake and seeking medical advice for recurrent problems. To me, that would be defensive medicine practices, and in the long run would prove to reduce morbidity, mortality and the cost of medical care.

Attempting to consider all possibilities by ordering additional tests and treatments or obtaining other opinions from specialist physicians should be labeled as comprehensive and thoughtful care by a physician and not the practice of defensive medicine. We need to rethink this issue.

• • •

I'M SORRY

It is well-known that the majority of medical malpractice claims filed against doctors, nurses and hospitals do not meet criteria needed to prove medical negligence.

In order to claim malpractice, it must be proven, to a degree of reasonable probability, that health care providers departed from accepted standards of care principles in their treatment of a patient and that this departure is directly linked to the cause of injury or death.

So why are there so many lawsuits? What drives many individuals who have sustained a bad medical outcome to file a lawsuit, however, is often a need to pay expensive medical bills and provide short and long-term care for an injury. However, there is a large group of patients who file lawsuits because they are angry.

Breakdown in communication between physician and patient following a bad outcome can have a profound effect with a patient feeling that their doctor does not care or that important information is being withheld.

Studies have confirmed that it is this breakdown in communication that often leads to a patient filing a lawsuit. Because of this, the medical profession has asked the question: how can doctors address this anger without implying guilt, and what can be done to avoid anger in the first place?

One suggestion is for doctors to sit down with their patient who has sustained a medical error or when an unanticipated clinical outcome occurs, even in the absence of mistakes, and say "I am sorry." Obviously, one problem with this approach has always been (similar to the Miranda rights) that "anything that you say can and will be used against you in a court of law."

In many instances, physicians are concerned that if they say to their patients, "I'm sorry" or express a similar sentiment of remorse, that this will be used against them in a medical malpractice case.

Interestingly, this "defend and deny" approach has actually led to lawsuits that might have otherwise been avoided and several states have passed legislation to address this concern.

In 2005 the Ohio General Assembly has recently passed H.B. 215, an act that prohibits the use of a doctor's apology or expression of sympathy as evidence of liability in a medical malpractice case. In other words, doctors who talk with patients or family members following a bad outcome do not have to worry about having what is said come back to haunt them.

The act states "all statements, affirmations, gestures, or conduct expressing apology, sympathy, commiseration, condolence, compassion, or a general sense of benevolence" is to be inadmissible and off-limits in issues brought up in medical malpractice litigation.

The Ohio law is patterned after Colorado's "I'm Sorry" law and was passed to create a layer of evidentiary protection for doctors so they can speak candidly with their patients and, it is hoped, to deter the filing of some potential malpractice claims. It is widely believed that offering an apology is extremely effective in reducing liability in cases when patients have had an unfortunate medical outcome.

Even when lawsuits are filed, it is also believed that an expression of condolence may aid in lower settlements. By offering an apology and condolences to a patient or family members, anger towards a physician can be significantly reduced or eliminated which can have a profound effect on a patient's desire to file a lawsuit.

At some prestigious hospitals such as Johns Hopkins and Dana-Farber Cancer Institute, policies have been adopted that encourage doctors to talk to patients and admit mistakes when they occur and offer an apology. Insurance companies have also begun teaching doctors how to discuss medical errors with patients, and certain guidelines have surfaced to help doctors in this approach.

Doctors need to take the initiative to contact the patient or family as soon as possible after a bad outcome since time allows feelings of anger to increase. Doctors need to have a good understanding of what happened and to not speculate in their discussions with patients and their families.

In addition, all questions should be openly and honestly answered and doctors should understand that apologizing or expressing condolences should not turn into finger pointing at others.

Doctors should keep in mind that, in many instances, it is only necessary to say, "I'm sorry" and patients should keep in mind that expressions of sympathy do not necessarily equate to admission of wrongdoing. Finally, doctors should discuss these issues with their risk management personnel, so that all involved members will be able to be on the same page.

Saying "I'm sorry" or expressing condolences is not a cure to avoid malpractice claims; however, it may create an environment in which a patient's understanding of what happened will be increased and anger defused. That certainly would be a good start.

• • •

BEDSIDE MANNERS

The few dozen first and second year medical students sat quietly and attentively as a nurse and I explained some of the important do's and don'ts of talking to patients about sensitive subjects. We were doing this in an educational session titled, "Dealing With Sensitive Subjects," and have found that it is very much appreciated by our medical school students.

These young students often have no idea how to go about informing patients of bad news or dealing with difficult, sensitive subjects such as death and dying, or how to talk to patients in a manner best suited to bring understanding and comfort.

In a *New York Times* article on the subject of talking about sensitive subjects to patients several years ago, Dr. Robert W. Blum, a pediatrician at the University of Minnesota School of Medicine, stated that, "We get very little training in dealing with these issues. As is true of people in general, we often do not know what to say."

Dr. Blum is not alone in his opinion. A Lewis-Harris poll of 230 physicians found that 61 percent stated they felt inadequately trained to properly communicate with their patients on sensitive subjects.

That is not good news and explains why many medical schools are trying to help young physicians learn how to handle those difficult moments such as when a parent needs to be told their child has a serious illness or has died, or when a patient has to be told of a bad outcome on a medical test.

Despite our efforts, however, we are not doing a good enough job. The results speak for themselves. A survey of 182 families with chronically sick or disabled children in Seattle and Minneapolis was conducted to assess how doctors handled sensitive situations.

The survey found that physicians still have a difficult time breaking bad news to patients. Important findings of the survey were that some doctors talk to the patient's family in an insensitive or dismissive manner, conveyed negative attitudes, or just did not respond to questions and concerns.

While most physicians appropriately deal with these issues, the fact that many do not is quite troubling. Guidelines exist on how to discuss bad news with patients. However, having guidelines is obviously not enough since one study revealed that only a third of doctors follow the majority of recommended guidelines.

When asked why they were not following these guidelines, some physicians reported that they did not have the time to talk to families, or that they were not heard properly. In fact, the vast majority of physicians described themselves as being available and supportive.

Obviously, one existing problem is that what is thought to be supportive by physicians is not necessarily considered supportive by the patient or family.

Clearly, those of us responsible for educating young doctors need to close this gap. One way to do this is through role playing, which is exactly what we do in our class at Vanderbilt Medical School.

Although each student needs to undergo thorough training on how to speak to patients about sensitive subjects, their personality and ability to demonstrate sensitivity and caring will ultimately determine how they respond to patients who are in crisis.

Young men and women of medicine need to learn through their own experiences as well as by observing older, more seasoned clinicians handle these situations properly.

While that may not completely solve the problem, it will at least be a start in helping those of us entrusted with being the bearer of bad news to do so in a clear, compassionate, supportive and caring manner.

・・・

MEN CRY, TOO

I have never understood why our society has made crying a gender issue. Why is it when a woman cries she is accepted, understood, and offered emotional support? Yet, when a man reveals his inner soul by shedding tears, the response is quite different.

As a young man I was told in both direct and indirect ways that big boys don't cry. It was a sign of weakness. When I entered medical school 40 years ago (95+% male students), that same message was loud and clear to those of us who were to become the next generation of American physicians.

Yet despite these negative attitudes and warnings against openly crying, at times I simply could not help myself and surrendered to my inner feelings and overflowing tear ducts. I had always felt it was a genetic trait because my father seemed to share this same trait.

I remember what happened to Senator Edmund Muskie when he wept at a press conference because a newspaper had made disparaging remarks about his wife while running for the 1972 Presidency. Neither the press nor the voters could accept his emotional response and, despite being a front-runner for the democratic ticket, his candidacy crumbled. Muskie's tears were too much for Americans to handle.

How times have changed! Since September 11, I have noticed a shift in societal response to male crying. Crying is no longer a sign a weakness.

When President George W. Bush revealed a rim of tears during one of his early responses to the terrorist attack, a nation felt comforted, not alarmed by his display of inner passion. And when many brave New York City firemen broke down during dozens of TV interviews, our nation was deeply moved and touched by their outward show of emotions.

I am not surprised. Men often cry at times of stress and crisis, however, until recently, they did so in private.

I first witnessed this dichotomy when, as a young physician in training, I helped a private physician care for a pregnant woman whose child died at the time of delivery and who, because of serious post delivery complications, also died. I could not hold back the tears as this patient's doctor explained to her waiting family what had happened in a very professional, stoic manner.

I couldn't believe anyone could be so detached and unemotional. However, when I retreated to what I thought was an empty lounge; I heard the muffled sounds of someone crying. It was the patient's physician. Believing that no one else was in the room, he had also broken down and was letting his emotions flow.

Years ago I read an article by Dr. Nancy R. Angoff in the *Piece of My Mind* section of the *Journal of the American Medical Association*. In it she noted that when she asked third year medical students if they ever cried during their clinical rotations, 133 of the 182 responded that they cried at least once, 30 had been on the verge of crying, and only 19 denied that they had cried.

The medical students did, however, worry about their crying, and often ran to bathrooms or stairwells to hide their emotions. They were concerned that other medical team members would be critical of their emotional overflow.

Fortunately, today's medical students (60% male) need not be so concerned about revealing their emotional side to the medical community. The medical profession, as well as society as a whole, no longer considers a man weak for showing his emotional side, even when tears glisten and run down his face.

This new public acceptance of support for crying men should be comforting to all of us. It is believed by many that much of the violent and aggressive behavior by males that we have witnessed in the past could be mollified and perhaps even lessened if our society were more accepting of men showing their true inner feelings during times of overwhelming stress.

September 11 changed much in our lives. One of those changes is the acceptance of men openly and unashamedly crying. Male tears reveal strength not weakness, compassion not fear, maturity not loss of control.

It seems we have finally come to the realization that crying is a healthy universal human emotion and not a gender issue.

• • •

BOUTIQUE MEDICINE

The first time I heard about MDVIP, I was having dinner with friends in Boca Raton, Florida. My friends were discussing two Boca Raton physicians who had started a unique type of practice where they planned to limit the number of their patients by charging an annual fee of $1500 per patient. This practice would enable physicians to offer VIP medical care.

To say the least, I was surprised to learn about this new approach to the practice of medicine. But before I offered my opinion, I knew I needed to do my homework on what I knew would become a very controversial subject.

I found that doctors in many cities had instituted this new type of practice called boutique or concierge medicine in response to increasing frustration over not having the time to dispense a personal and thorough type of medical care.

In Boca Raton, Boston, Phoenix and Seattle several medical groups began significantly limiting the number of patients in their practice, from thousands to 600 in Boca Raton, 300 in Boston and 50 in Seattle, while charging annual fees of $1500-$20,000. Boutique medicine is currently being considered in New York, California, Illinois, Texas, Maryland and Virginia.

Patients accepting this type of additional charge are told that they can expect amenities that they have been unable to receive in the past.

While these amenities vary from practice to practice, they include: same day appointments, physician availability (24/7/365), comprehensive annual physical exams, email and cell phone access to the doctor, internet access to medical records, annual nutrition and physical fitness assessments in patient's homes or health clubs, home visits, private reception and examination areas replete with heated towel racks, marble showers and personally monogrammed robes and accompaniment to emergency rooms and referred specialist's offices.

Physicians who practice this "membership fee" type of medicine argue that by charging an entry fee they can have a limited and small number of patients, and thus be able to spend much more time with their patients at each medical encounter.

Physicians who have begun this type of practice insist they are not necessarily making more money but rather are finally practicing the kind of medicine they had always hoped to practice. Gone are the huge numbers of patients in the waiting room, the limited time spent with each patient and the inability to attend to their entire needs.

While I can understand why some doctors in this country are resorting to this type of practice, I am saddened that our health care system has come to this. I am saddened to think that we have come to a time in medicine where patients have to pay a substantial membership fee to get what many of us went into medicine to give as a routine practice.

Boutique or concierge practices may be a solution for an individual doctor and wealthy patients, but it is not a solution for our society.

If large numbers of physicians were to limit their practices to only those who can afford these additional thousands of dollars, who will be left to take care of the many who cannot pay? What will this say about our compassionate profession?

We do not need a medical system in which physicians charge extra for compassionate, personal, thorough and expert medical care. We need an environment in which our health care system provides funds that allows physicians to treat *every* patient with compassionate, personal, thorough and expert medical care.

• • •

THE VALUE OF NURSES

While I have been given much good advice in my lifetime, one of the best was given by my chief resident when I began an internship in Surgery in 1965.

"Do yourself a favor, Frank, make sure you go to each of the nurses on the floors you will be working, introduce yourself, let them know you would appreciate any helpful points they might be able to give you on how to take good care of your patients, and let them know that you understand they have considerably more experience than you and that you are eager to learn from their experience and wisdom. Show them that you respect them as nurses." How right he was!

While it took a week to fulfill that advice, it was well worth the time and effort. Not only did I learn an incredible amount of information that helped me take better care of my patients, I also noticed that many of my fellow interns who did not take this advice were more frequently awakened in the middle of the night than I was in order to take care of matters that could have easily been attended to the next morning.

It seemed that the better the doctors treated the nurses, the better the nurses treated the doctors.

Nurses are, quite frankly, the backbone of health care. While physicians play an incredibly important and critical role in overall health care, nurses are often the ones who help carry out that care, point out problems along the way, stick around to calm fears, help explain matters and bring peace and comfort to patients and families, often after everyone else has left the scene.

In Intensive Care Units, it is the nurse who knows how to monitor all the vital signs of a critically ill patient, understands how to set up and use extremely complicated instruments used to obtain these vital signs and is there by the bedside 24 hours a day, seven days a week, updating physicians on the condition of patients.

In operating rooms, it is the nurse who first enters the room and readies it for the soon-to-be-admitted patient in need of extensive and often complicated lifesaving surgery. Machines are turned on and checked for accuracy while operating packs are laid out and made ready for use by physicians.

Studies have demonstrated that there are direct links between a shortage of nurses and patient complications. Serious medical complications in hospitals such as pneumonia, upper gastrointestinal bleeding, shock and cardiac arrest occur up to 9% more often when there are low levels of nurse staffing on hospital floors.

As patient advocates, nurses watch over their patients and help avoid errors as well as alert physicians to early signs and symptoms of trouble.

It has been said that a chain is as strong as its weakest link. Nurses are a strong link in a lengthy chain that helps provide health care to patients in doctor's offices, hospitals, and outpatient facilities all across America. That is why I am so concerned about the future of the nursing profession in this country.

Simply put, there is an emerging nurse shortage in this country that many are calling a health care crisis. The combination of an increase in the elderly, an increase in chronic diseases and an aging nursing population is creating real concern for the ability of our health care system to adequately take care of its patients now and especially in the future.

Studies reveal that only half as many women today select a career in nursing as compared to 25 years ago. Since 1973 there has been a 40% decrease in the number of college freshmen who indicate that nursing was even among some of their top career choices.

While the number of entry-level nurses increased by 90,000 in 2003 (the highest level reported since 1987), the current percentage of working nurses over the age of 40 is high and increasing. Currently, approximately 60% of nurses are over 40 years of age.

Studies have shown that the average age of nurses is increasing at double the rate of all other professions in America and that the percentage and total number of nurses under the age of 30 has dropped.

The recent rise in the number of registered nurses entering the job market is due, in part, to older nurses returning to work on a part-time basis and to the import of foreign trained nurses. Even with these additional nurses, experts agree that nursing shortages will significantly increase over the next decade, and that this shortage will cripple the entire health care system.

It is projected that by 2010, 40% of working nurses will be over the age of 50, and by 2020 the number of available nurses will be below requirement levels, with all of this occurring just as the first of the 76 million baby boomers begin to require increased health care.

With the current nationwide shortage of nurses being in the range of 10%, it is estimated that by 2020, we will need 2.8 million full-time nurses to help take care of our patients, yet there will only be 2.2 million available.

The most prominent factor in this evolving nursing shortage is today's increased opportunity for women to choose other career paths that formerly were not open to women. Medicine, law and business are now openly and equally available to either sex and, while there is still some inequity in pay, women are flocking to non-nursing careers.

There are, however, other troubling reasons for a lackluster interest in nursing: lack of respect of nurses by physicians and health care administrators and difficult working conditions.

What then can be done to reverse this impending health care crisis? Here are a few suggestions: make a career in nursing more appealing to young women (and men) by increasing salaries, improving working conditions, especially for an older nursing population, allowing for an increase in nurse autonomy in the workplace, and making tuition benefit scholarships and loan re-payment programs available to nurses who want to advance their education.

In addition, train medical students, physicians in training, and practicing physicians to give those who have chosen nursing as their profession the same respect they do their physician colleagues.

While the current nursing shortages have created increased interest for young women and men to apply to nursing school, it has been reported that thousands of nursing school applicants have been turned away because of a shortage of nursing faculty.

It seems clear, that nursing education programs will have to find a way to overcome capacity problems in order to expand and meet the growing demands of more nurses in the workforce and that faculty positions will need to become much more attractive.

Without good nursing care, patients are often doomed to less than optimal outcomes. Without nurses, hospital functions will cease, beds will have to remain empty and hospitals will close. We must not let this happen.

· · ·

DOCTORS AND THE MEDIA

An article in the *Journal of the American Medical Association,* headlined "Medical Researchers and the Media," brought back some very powerful memories for me.

The authors of this study were interested in obtaining the opinion of medical scientists regarding their experience with the news media following the publication of their scientific reports in two of our country's most prestigious medical journals the *Journal of the American Medical Association* and the *New England Journal of Medicine.*

What they found did not surprise me. Medical researchers had positive attitudes toward the press, with 86% reporting that news reports based on their studies were accurate and 44% responding they felt media coverage would help them achieve their overall professional goals.

In addition, these physician/scientists stated that media coverage improved the image of the profession, imparted research information to the professional community and allowed the public to better understand their work.

Times certainly have changed. The father of medicine, Hippocrates, exhorted physicians to avoid activities that "savor or fuss or show," and in 1905, the noted physician Sir William Osler cautioned doctors not to "dally with the Delilah of the press." He warned that to communicate with the press could undermine the confidence of their colleagues.

Even as late as 1973, most physicians had a very negative view of doctors who openly communicated their work with the press. I should know.

Returning to Nashville after seven years of training in obstetrics and gynecology, I began performing a new female sterilization procedure at Vanderbilt called laparoscopic tubal ligation. This rather simple procedure allowed women to undergo a quick and safe operation for permanent sterilization without major surgery and without the need for overnight hospitalization or an extended recovery period as was required with an open abdominal surgical procedure.

This process, now routinely performed by gynecologists and surgeons for many other abdominal procedures, was in its infancy in the early 1970s and was a new and exciting procedure.

Performing approximately six of these on an outpatient basis every Friday morning at Vanderbilt, the news spread quickly throughout Nashville. Not surprisingly, a reporter from the *Tennessean* called me one day asking questions concerning this new technique. The following morning a front page article appeared on this innovative surgery for women with my direct quotes.

For the next few days the phones in my office did not stop ringing. Women all over middle Tennessee wanted to know how they could learn more about this new procedure. One phone call, however, was of a different nature.

The Nashville Academy of Medicine's Ethics Committee wanted to meet with me at their next meeting. They were concerned about the *Tennessean* article and wanted a face-to-face confrontation.

Only thirty-two years of age and at Vanderbilt University Hospital for less than a year, I was apprehensive to say the least. The events of that meeting can best be summarized by saying I received a slap on my wrist and a warning: *stop peddling your wares to the press. Doctors in Nashville do not do such things.*

At the time I felt the Ethics Committee lacked vision in their views and time has now certainly vindicated my thinking on this matter.

Today, hospitals have Public Relations departments to keep the written and electronic press well informed of every new, innovative and exciting advance in medicine coming out of their institutions. Our media is filled with accounts of scientific studies and physician opinions, as well as countless other human interest stories and ethical dilemmas found in the medical community.

I think today Hippocrates would agree our society is better off with these new attitudes by physicians and medical institutions towards the press.

Patients are now better informed and more able to make difficult decisions in health related matters. The article on medical researchers' opinions of the media has certainly indicated that times have changed, and for the better.

• • •

ETHICS OF MULTIPLE BIRTHS

The incredible delivery in Iowa in 1997 of seemingly healthy two to three pound septuplets born at almost 31 weeks' gestation, brought back vivid memories of a set of quintuplets I helped deliver in 1987. That amazingly rare delivery also made national news.

Unfortunately, because they were delivered at 24 weeks, four babies died of problems related to their extreme prematurity. Only the first born, Stephen Hawkins, survived. Thankfully, today Stephen is a normal, healthy child.

I vividly remember the tension, joy and excitement of the Hawkins' delivery as each baby tumbled out of their mother's womb. I also remember the sadness, as one by one, four small, tiny and fragile babies died.

And so, while I was happy for the McCaugheys' good fortune in delivering seven surviving children, at the same time I was worried and concerned that because of their story, many Americans may be lulled into a false sense of security and hope concerning the outcome of multiple pregnancies.

While other animals routinely deliver multiple offspring, the human uterus is made for only one child at a time. The complications of more than one fetus in the uterus are well-known to those of us in the health care profession.

All too often, because of a high incidence of premature birth, the outcome of multiple pregnancy is unfortunately tragic. Premature babies, who do survive depending on their gestational age, often have serious lifelong complications, including cerebral palsy, visual problems, chronic lung disease, learning disabilities and hearing loss, to name just a few.

Those of us entrusted to care for patients with multiple pregnancies have our hands full. Because of in-vitro fertilization and other effective medications to induce ovulation, the incidence of twins in this country has doubled, and the incidence of triplets has risen significantly. At one point a few years ago, I had three patients with a triplet gestation, something unheard of years ago.

An average infertile couple, therefore, needs to understand that by going through the many processes available in an effort to become pregnant, their chance of multiple birth is significantly elevated. They must decide in advance if they truly want to expose themselves to that possibility, because with that choice comes another difficult decision.

That decision is the selective abortion of one or more fetuses in hopes of improving pregnancy outcome for the remaining fetuses. Unfortunately, because many couples like the McCaugheys are unwilling to accept selective abortion as an alternative, they are forced to go through the multiple pregnancy with all its probable complications.

Doctors have an ethical responsibility to discuss all this with infertile couples in advance of treatment. While twins and triplets usually have a better outcome than higher number of multiple births, the fact is even these pregnancies can have serious and lifelong complications. Add to all this the ingredients of financial, emotional and physical costs, and it becomes clear that this is an important issue for many Americans.

Having raised three children, one at a time, I cannot imagine what the McCaugheys have had to go through these past years. I hope they have found the strength and courage to handle the new and multiple responsibilities as they are confronted with them.

I also hope that as we are continuously updated on this successful multiple birth pregnancy outcome, we keep in mind that good outcomes are rare exceptions. Bringing more than one or two fetuses at a time into the world is not only difficult and complicated; it is often dangerous as well.

• • •

WHAT TO DO

Except for one important fact, my two pregnant patients were totally different. One was an unmarried 16-year-old, the mother of a one-year-old and living with her mother on welfare. The other was a 42-year-old married lawyer, who had a long-standing history of infertility and who had finally gotten pregnant by an expensive and highly technical process known as in-vitro fertilization.

Both shared a serious and potentially life-threatening condition for their unborn. Both were 23 weeks pregnant and in premature labor.

A full-term pregnancy is reached at 37 weeks of gestation, therefore 23 weeks was extremely early. Fortunately, of the four million births each year in this country, only approximately 20,000 babies are born at 23 to 25 weeks of pregnancy. Unfortunately, these 20,000 babies encounter tremendous loss of life and serious lifelong handicaps if survival does occur.

The emotional heartache for parents, dealing with these extremely premature babies is difficult to describe and the cost to parents and society is often overwhelming. Helping such a small baby survive in our modern neonatal intensive care unit today costs approximately $2,000 each day. With hospitalizations running into months, bills of a quarter of a million dollars are not unusual.

As I walked into the rooms of each of these patients, I knew my task was to explain the obstetric dilemma each was in and to impart important information on survival and long-term outcome should these babies be delivered this early. I also realized that I must counsel both so as not to influence each with my own personal bias.

Based on reliable scientific information, I carefully explained that a baby born at 23 weeks gestation will have no more than a 15% (or 1 in 7) chance of long-term survival and that survival will be associated with severe abnormalities 98% of the time. If my patients could gain just one week without delivering, the survival rate for their newborn would change significantly.

Delivering at 24 weeks, babies have an approximately 50% chance of survival and a 1 in 5 chance of surviving without major handicaps. If we could somehow delay delivery two additional weeks, these babies would do even better since 80% of babies born at 25 weeks survive, and 70% of those surviving would do so without major long-term problems.

My patients, however, were far advanced in their premature labor. Because of this, both would require intensive and expensive treatment in our labor and delivery suite, and receive potent medications with multiple potential serious side effects in an attempt to stop their labor for a short period of time.

Both would require bed rest, separation from home as well as constant monitoring of fetal heart rate, uterine contractions and maternal vital signs. Because both babies were breech, a cesarean section would also need to be considered to avoid birth-trauma.

After discussing all this with both potential parents involved, I wondered if my advice should be different. Knowing the 16-year-old would have the opportunity to conceive again, should I encourage her to refrain from treatment thereby allowing her baby to deliver at 23 weeks resulting in probable death?

And what about my 42-year-old patient? This would probably be her only chance for motherhood. Should I encourage her to do everything possible to save her child's life?

My two patients presented vastly different social issues, yet my approach to both could not differ. The equal distribution of the burdens and benefits of medical care, demanded of me by the ethical principle of social justice, helped direct me in the care of these two very different patients.

Despite their differences, both patients asked me to do what I could to prolong the pregnancy and help their child survive. Both delivered within 2 weeks and both children, while undergoing extensive care in our newborn intensive care unit, survived.

While I do not know what happened to these children, I do know I did the right thing.

• • •

WHEN LIFE BEGINS

How one comes to an opinion on the subject of abortion often depends on when one considers life to begin. If one takes a position that abortion should not be performed after life begins, then the answer to the question, "when does life begin" obviously has considerable impact on an individual's stand on the subject of abortion.

As an obstetrician for over 35 years, and having been involved in the abortion issue for at least that long I have been asked many times, "when does life begin?" It is an important question to ask, however, it is not an easy one to answer.

Because of varying philosophical, ethical, social, moral, religious, political, legal, and medical opinions, no one answer satisfies everyone in our heterogeneous society as the one and only true answer.

There can be as many as five different answers given to the question of when life begins. The first is that life begins when egg and sperm unite in fertilization while the second is that life begins when a pregnancy test becomes positive, which can occur as early as a day after the dividing cells of a fertilized egg implants into the uterus (approximately 7 days after fertilization). The third answer is that life begins when fetal brain wave activity first occurs (approximately 12 weeks from a woman's first day of her last menstrual period).

There are those who believe life begins at that gestational age when a fetus has a reasonable chance of survival outside its mother's womb (currently 24 weeks), while finally, there is a fifth answer that life begins at the time of delivery.

Each of these five answers presents significant logical, medical, ethical, social or legal problems. Consider the logical problem that life begins when egg unites with sperm. Understanding the fact that each fertilized egg has the potential to split into a separate embryo (identical twins) up to the 14th day after conception, how are we to define the status of the initial conception prior to splitting?

Jim Holt, a New York writer, attempted to resolve this issue in a 1992 *New Republic* magazine article. Making a logical and philosophical point that the newly formed twins cannot be equal to the original conception, nor can they be equal to each other (even identical twins are not exactly alike), and that if the original conception is neither of the twins, then it cannot be considered a person.

Since separation of the fertilized egg can take place up to 14 days, the embryo until that time "lacks any property that would make it one definite human being. In Aristotle's terms, it lacks a soul. It is not a person but the source of an indeterminate number of potential persons much like a collection of sperm and eggs."

Using the definition of life beginning with a positive pregnancy test would effectively make all abortions illegal. While that may satisfy many anti-choice advocates, it would not satisfy the majority of Americans who believe abortion should be kept legally available.

In addition, it is highly likely that if our society were to ban all abortions tomorrow, the overall number of abortions would not be significantly reduced, while maternal mortality and morbidity would be significantly elevated by an increase in illegal abortions.

Because legal and medical practices define death as loss of all brain function, using life's beginning with the first presence of brain function at approximately 12 weeks does make some sense. Using that answer, however, would eliminate the medical use of abortion in situations of maternal illness or fetal abnormalities after 12 weeks.

The fourth answer as to when life begins is currently widely accepted. While allowing abortion up to the point of viability presents moral, ethical and religious issues, it does satisfy the current legal climate, as well as meeting medical needs of our society.

The fifth answer offends many individuals and presents huge ethical concerns, but is included here because Roe vs. Wade's decision makes it legal for doctors to perform abortions well into the third trimester. Fortunately, only a few individuals believe that life begins only at delivery.

So there you have it. Pick your answer and take your stand. Perhaps my father had the best answer of all. When asked once when he believed life began, he responded "when my son got into medical school."

• • •

ABORTION AND GESTATIONAL LIMITS

It has been almost a third of a century since the Supreme Court ruled on Roe vs. Wade and made abortion legal in this country.

During this time, there have been incredible medical advances that have prolonged life expectancy, cured cancers, increased survival rates for AIDS patients, reduced the suffering of dozens of serious chronic illnesses, as well as significantly increasing the survival rates of small premature babies.

In 1973, a premature baby born at 24 weeks (counting from the woman's last menstrual period), had virtually no chance of survival after delivery. Today, that same baby has a 50% chance of survival. Even at 28 weeks of pregnancy, few newborns were able to survive while, today, 90% of 28 week premature babies survive.

Clearly, some things have dramatically changed. Modern neonatal intensive care units have, with advances in ventilation support, drugs, diagnostic tools and lung surfactant treatment, dramatically increased survival rates, while reducing morbidity of very small premature babies.

The Supreme Court's ruling, which defined what was permissible by each trimester of pregnancy, is no longer as defendable as it once was. Considering each trimester to be divided into 13 week blocks, it becomes obvious that by the end of the second trimester (24 to 26 weeks), the fetus has a significant chance of survival outside its mother's womb (50 to 75%) and therefore, should be considered viable.

Certainly, by the third trimester (27 to 40 weeks) abortion, which is defined as a procedure in which a physician intends to deliver a stillborn fetus, should no longer be permissible.

Some pro-choice activists claim that abortion should be available even at these later gestational ages in order to save the life or health of a woman or if the fetus is seriously malformed. While that may sound reasonable to some, it misses the point.

In a case when the life or health of a mother is in jeopardy, and her fetus has reached a reasonable chance of survival outside the womb and therefore viable, physicians can deliver that child by either a Cesarean section or induction of labor without compromising the mother's health any more than by performing an abortion. By doing this, the child will at least have a chance of survival. Physicians currently do this thousands of times each year.

If the fetus is 24 weeks or more and has a serious malformation which is incompatible with life, then a pre-term delivery process will result in a child who will die naturally after delivery. Thus, there is no need for a physician to deliver the fetus stillborn. This occurs, for example, with anencephalic fetuses (fetuses born without the top of their brain and skull) or Potter's syndrome (the absence of both fetal kidneys).

On the other hand when the fetus is 24 weeks or more and has a malformation or defect that is compatible with life, such as Down syndrome or spina bifida, most physicians throughout this country do not believe it appropriate to perform an abortion. Because virtually all major malformations and genetic disorders can be diagnosed prior to 20 weeks of pregnancy, women with these problems can usually be given the option of abortion well before the 24 week stage of pregnancy has been reached.

States need to address the constitutionality of each bill it attempts to pass to establish gestational age limits with abortion. However, each state needs to also keep in mind that times have changed and that a fetus is more likely to survive in the late second trimester than it ever was when Roe vs. Wade was upheld by the Supreme Court in 1973.

The public needs to understand these facts and issues. It is medically, morally and ethically reasonable to prohibit abortion after viability of a fetus has been reached. Today, that is 24 weeks of gestation. By prohibiting abortion after this gestational age, no slippery slope will be stumbled upon, no mother will suffer loss of life or health and no fetus with a lethal anomaly will survive.

The one thing that will happen, however, is that our society will be doing the right thing for the right reasons.

• • •

ABORTION FOR GENDER SELECTION

The married couple sitting in my office was intelligent, straightforward and sincere. "If it is a girl, we want an abortion" the husband explained, his wife shaking her head in agreement. The couple from India, in this country on a training grant, while very happy with their two girls, was adamant that their third and last child must be a boy. "Could you help us?" they asked.

It was not the first time that I have had couples request my help in diagnosing the sex of a fetus with the intention of aborting their child if it was the "wrong sex." I understood the problem.

Our American culture differs from that of other countries. In several countries, such as India and China, having a male child is of the utmost importance. It is a son who will carry on the family name, inherit family wealth, care for parents as they age, and light the father's funeral pyres (helping place the soul at peace for eternity).

On the other hand, when girls grow up and marry, they require a dowry, which is given to the groom's family, and then leave home to join the family of her new husband.

When parents grow old and need financial or other types of assistance, it is a son and not a daughter, who assumes this responsibility. Because of this, couples feel as if they need at least one male child, and, consequently, many couples in these countries decide to abort female fetuses.

The problem with gender selection has become so acute in India that sex determination testing was outlawed in 1994 because of significant changes in female to male ratios.

The number of females per 1000 males in India had dropped from 962 in 1981 to 927. In certain affluent parts of India that number has declined to an astonishing 793 girls for every 1000 boys! (In the U.S. it is 1029 females to 1000 males.)

Despite the 1994 law prohibiting sex determination, not much has changed. Women throughout India can still obtain an ultrasound examination in the second trimester of their pregnancy and obtain an abortion if they are carrying a female fetus.

To date, no one in India has been legally accused of violating this law. Ultrasound machines are often moved from village to village throughout India to offer sex determination for concerned pregnant patients.

My patient, however, was in America and confronting a different set of cultural values when she and her husband requested an early diagnosis of fetal sex. I explained to the couple that I could not help them because I would not perform a medical test merely in order to determine fetal gender, thereby allowing for a decision of whether to have an abortion.

I also explained that I would not abort their pregnancy on the basis of selecting gender for cultural and social reasons.

Just as women in this country have the right to choose or not choose abortion, I also have a right (based on the ethical principal of autonomy) to choose whether or not to participate in helping a patient carry out that choice.

I wonder what will happen someday when those countries which elevate the value of males, suddenly find they have significantly more males than females. Perhaps when young men cannot find enough young women to marry, those countries encouraging gender selection will take a long, hard look at enforcing laws which prevent such selection as the sole criteria for abortion.

Maybe, someday, in those countries, it will be the girl's family who receives a dowry.

• • •

PARTIAL BIRTH ABORTION

Growing up in the Bible Belt of the South, I am accustomed to hearing that important religious writings contain answers for most of life's difficult questions. While some may disagree with this statement, I have found that on the issue of partial birth abortion, the Talmud, though written thousands of years ago, may have many right answers for our society today.

The Talmud, a text written by ancient rabbis approximately 2000 years ago and attempts to answer questions not addressed in the Old Testament, states that, "If a woman is in hard labor (and her life is in danger), they cut up the fetus within her womb and remove it limb by limb, because her life takes precedence over that of the fetus. But if the greater part was already born, they may not touch him, for one may not set aside one person's life for that of another" (Mishna Ohalot 7:6).

This important religious document makes clear that one is designated a person only after "the greater part (of the fetus) was already born." Religious scholars two millenniums ago seemed to speak to us today about the controversy of partial birth abortion and would strongly condemn such a procedure.

President George W. Bush signed into law a ban on a procedure known as partial birth abortion. This law criminalizes an abortion technique for the first time in history and has caused considerable controversy.

Many abortion rights advocates argue that this law puts us on a slippery slope towards overturning Roe vs. Wade, while abortion opponents believe that it is a monument to the sanctity of life.

The law states that "the term partial birth abortion means an abortion in which the person performing the abortion deliberately and intentionally vaginally delivers a living fetus until any part of the fetal trunk past the navel is outside the body of the mother, for the purpose of performing an overt act that the person knows will kill the partially delivered living fetus."

In other words, once the greater portion of the child is outside the mother's body, a physician may not perform any procedure that would lead to its death. Sound familiar?

Americans have long been conflicted over the subject of abortion. Statistics, however, indicate that the vast majority wish to keep abortions legal, safe and rare while at the same time wanting the process to have certain limitations.

Although most Americans label themselves as either pro-life or pro-choice, many in both these groups add a "but" to that label. That "but" contains issues such as parental consent, gestational age limits, a 24 hour waiting period, limited Federal Government payments for abortion, and a ban on partial birth abortion.

On this latter issue, it seems that most Americans are in agreement that partial birth abortion, usually performed after 20 weeks of gestation, should be banned.

The partial birth abortion debate caused some erosion of support for abortion rights. In 1995, when the controversy first surfaced, 31% of Americans supported a woman's right to choose abortion under any circumstance.

After three years of bitter debate, that support dropped to 23%. Today, that support is even lower. It seems Americans are turned off to extreme positions taken by those who support partial birth abortion.

A relatively recent Gallup poll found that the percentage of Americans who consider themselves pro-life rose from 33% to 43% over the past few years, and the percentage of those who consider themselves pro-choice declined from 56% to 48% during that same time period.

While there is a definitive shift away from pro-choice support, polls also reveal that Americans still favor keeping abortion legal. Over the past few years, the percentage of those who favor outlawing all abortions has not changed. It remains at approximately 20%, with the remaining 80% indicating that they want abortion to be legal, under any circumstance or legal in some circumstances.

However, if the pro-choice movement is to continue to maintain support of the majority of Americans, it will have to rethink how it addresses a number of critical issues surrounding abortion, including partial birth abortion.

First, it will need to defend abortion rights within a moral framework. The pro-choice movement needs to openly admit that abortion is a death and that the consequences to many women are real and significant. They cannot minimize the value of life, even though they support abortion rights.

Morality surrounds the abortion issues so much that when asked if abortion was a matter between a woman, her doctor, her family, her conscience and her God, 72% of Americans agreed. However, when asked the same question without using the word God or conscience, only 42% agreed.

While there are 1.2 million abortions performed each year in this country, less than a few thousand partial birth abortions are performed with only a handful of doctors performing the procedure.

The issue is more political than medical, since there is never a medical indication for this type of abortion. By refusing to support a ban on partial birth abortion, the pro-choice movement is losing American support.

Supporting a ban on this type of abortion will not, however, be enough to reassure Americans that the movement is not in the hands of extremists.

I believe that pro-choice organizations should also support one parent consent (with a judicial bypass) for minors; a 24 hour waiting period; a ban on most Federal funding; and gestational age limits on abortion once viability has been achieved (24 weeks from last menstrual period). These measures will, to some degree, reassure Americans that the pro-choice movement is willing to display compromise, common sense and compassion.

It may be true that we are on a slippery slope because of this first ban on an abortion procedure. However, I think that we could have avoided this slope by a united condemnation of an extreme procedure that offends so many Americans on both sides of the abortion debate and is contrary to religious doctrine written 2000 years ago.

The United States Supreme Court will, undoubtedly, review this new law. Based on their decision to not support such a ban passed by the state of Nebraska in 2000, it is almost certain that this ban signed into law by our President, will also be overturned. I think that will be a shame. I believe, on this issue, our religious scholars got it right many years ago.

• • •

EMERGENCY CONTRACEPTION

There was a time, not very long ago, when buying condoms in a drugstore was one of the most emotionally traumatic moments a young man could experience.

Approaching the pharmacist's counter, often with several customers standing around, and asking for a package of condoms was not only embarrassing, it was also very intimidating. This certainly prevented many young men from obtaining condoms.

Times certainly have changed. Condoms are now stocked on shelves in aisles along with aspirin, vitamins, and other drugstore items, so those embarrassing and intimidating moments with a pharmacist are now bypassed.

What was done to make condom sales for males more accessible and acceptable should now be done for women. If our society is truly interested in reducing unwanted pregnancies and abortions, one good way to accomplish this goal is to make emergency contraception (also known as the morning after pill) more accessible.

Emergency contraception is not new. A Canadian in 1974 reported that women who had unprotected intercourse and took a high-dose regimen of birth control pills within three days prevented approximately 75% of pregnancies that might be expected without such treatment.

Slow to gain acceptance in this country, emergency contraception has been proven to be quite effective. Approximately 8 out of every 100 women having one episode of unprotected intercourse during ovulation time will become pregnant without emergency contraception treatment, while only 2 out of 100 will become pregnant with emergency contraception medication.

The Allen Guttmacher Institute estimates that emergency contraception prevented 50,000 abortions in 2000. That figure could reach hundreds of thousands if information of this technique to prevent unwanted pregnancies was made more available to

American women, and if emergency contraception medication could be sold over-the-counter, as it is in Europe.

One company currently manufactures Food and Drug Administration approved emergency contraception medication. Plan B (Levonorgestrel), when taken within 72 hours of unprotected intercourse and repeated in 12 hours, at a cost of $20 to $30 a treatment, can prevent an unwanted pregnancy. The manufacturer of Plan B applied to the FDA to obtain over-the-counter approval; however, the FDA has, for the time being, turned down their request.

It is critical that women be able to walk into a pharmacy, buy emergency contraception medication over-the-counter, and begin treatment as soon as possible after an unprotected sexual encounter. Waiting to see a doctor to obtain emergency contraception medication will not work for most women.

The most effective reduction in pregnancy rates is noted when the medication is taken within 24 hours. Although currently California, Alaska, Washington, New Mexico, Maine and Hawaii have laws that allow pharmacists to prescribe emergency contraception medication, as happened with condoms, the intimidation factor (especially for teenagers) is a deterrent.

The morning after pill is used mostly by women 19 to 29 years of age and has been shown not to result in indiscriminate use. Making emergency contraception available to 540 women in one study resulted in only ten women using it more than one time and in another study of 2,117 young women, aged 15-24, it was noted that easier access to emergency contraception did not lead to an increase of sexual activity, nor did it compromise usual contraceptive methods.

The problem is that emergency contraception is controversial. Although emergency contraception works primarily by interfering with ovulation and therefore preventing fertilization (egg and sperm uniting), it is possible that in some cases it may work by preventing implantation of an already fertilized egg into the uterus.

With no absolute method to prove if this latter event is the mechanism by which emergency contraception works (since without implantation pregnancy tests will not become positive), some anti-choice groups maintain that emergency contraception pills cause an abortion and, therefore, will not approve its use. Some opponents also incorrectly confuse emergency contraception medication with RU486, a drug used for the purpose of causing abortion.

Approximately half of all American women between the ages of 15 to 44 have at least one unplanned pregnancy at sometime in their lives.

With half of the 6 million pregnancies each year in this country estimated to occur in women who had not planned a pregnancy, and with over one million abortions being performed each year, it is time to help women prevent an unwanted pregnancy during those times when condoms break, spermicidal tablets do not melt, birth control pills are missed, or when couples use no contraception during an unplanned and perhaps unexpected sexual encounter.

If emergency contraception medication is approved someday for over-the-counter sales, women all across America will have something they can do to avoid an unplanned pregnancy and will be able to obtain that remedy as easily as men can now purchase condoms.

• • •

MORALITY AND THE PHARMACIST

I have always envied those who could respond to difficult issues with a black or white response. On controversial issues I often seem to find the gray and, therefore, have considerable difficulty in being dogmatic and absolute.

I find that there usually are two relatively strong positions on most controversial issues with those who articulate one side or the other often making excellent points. Such is the case on the recent difficult issue of pharmacists who refuse to dispense birth control medication (or other medicines) to patients because of moral or religious convictions that these medications could cause an abortion.

It was reported in 2005 that there were approximately 180 reports of pharmacists throughout the United States who had refused to fill prescriptions written by doctors for birth control or emergency contraception medication on the grounds that filling these prescriptions would violate their moral and ethical principles.

Despite the fact that there have been no such reports in Tennessee in the past nine years, legislation is being offered by our legislators that would permit the 5,200 pharmacists in Tennessee to refuse to fill any prescription that violates their ethical or religious principles.

While one could argue that our government cannot and should not attempt to legislate morality, it is equally true that one should not dispense morality at a drug store. Here comes the gray.

In my field of Obstetrics, doctors in practice or training are given an option to refuse to participate in the process of performing an abortion. However, we make it clear that if an Obstetrician-Gynecologist will not perform an abortion, they must refer their patient to a doctor who would.

This process works well for doctor and patient alike. However, being turned away by a pharmacist who may be the only one in town, may present considerable hardship on patients throughout our state.

But if a pharmacist is truly conflicted about dispensing a drug which they believe may induce an abortion and therefore goes against their moral belief, what are they to do? And how will they deal with similar issues?

Will some pharmacists refuse to dispense erectile dysfunction medication to men who are known to be gay, HIV positive or merely single? What if a pharmacist is told that the requested birth control medication is not for contraception, but rather for menstrual cramps or acne? Will that make a difference?

How will a pharmacist know whether emergency contraception (which delays ovulation and can prevent an unwanted pregnancy in three out of four instances) is being requested because of rape or carelessness?

What about the sale of condoms, diaphragms, spermicidal jelly or creams? Where is all this dispensing of morality by pharmacists going to lead us? Most states have left these kinds of decisions to pharmacists to decide and most state pharmacy leaders have stated that they want to keep it that way.

It turns out that the American Pharmacy Association has a policy that allows pharmacists to refuse filling medications but also adds that these pharmacists must call another pharmacist, either in that store or somewhere nearby, to take care of the prescription. So, I asked myself: Why are there politicians in Tennessee who want to pass such a law? Why do they want to open Pandora's Box?

In seems apparent to me that this and similar laws are attempts to chip away at abortion and contraception rights. I object to this intrusion of patient rights and hope the Tennessee legislature will have the backbone to not pass this law.

I believe that sincere pharmacists have a right to refuse filling any prescription that violates their religious beliefs. But, I also believe that they have an ethical duty to make sure that the patient can get his or her medication filled by another pharmacist in that store or one nearby.

It should also be required that pharmacists must prominently place notices in their pharmacy acknowledging that they retain the right to refuse to honor certain prescriptions, so that potential customers know in advance and can go elsewhere.

Refusing to fill certain prescriptions could backfire if enough potential customers got together to show their displeasure by boycotting all merchandise at that store. If pharmacists have a right to fill or not fill a prescription, consumers also have a right to buy or not buy from them. If nothing else these pharmacists might be forced to always have someone available who will fill any prescription.

I have respect for those who train to become pharmacists. They go to school a long time, work hard and fill a very important role in our daily lives.

However, if pharmacy is their calling, then they will need to address this important issue before entering the field. If they still chose this profession, then they need to make sure that as they exercise their moral and religious principles, they also understand that patients who are sent to them also have a right to exercise theirs.

Which brings me back to the gray area: pharmacists have a right to refuse but also have a responsibility to make sure their clients are able to easily fill prescriptions.

Perhaps this would be a good time for the Food and Drug Administration to approve over-the-counter sale of emergency contraception and therefore by-pass the pharmacist altogether. It is also a good time to cool the rhetoric, dismiss this legislation that is not needed and let market factors and doing the right thing dictate actions.

• • •

OREGON AND PHYSICIAN-ASSISTED SUICIDE

While I have maintained a vigorous and persistent objection to physician-assisted suicide over the past 30 years, I must admit that Oregon's Death with Dignity law, which has allowed physicians to legally participate in helping patients die over the past 6 years, has been surprisingly instructive.

To begin with, the number of patients requesting medication that would cause death has been small, and the number of patients actually taking the lethal medication has been even smaller.

Since 1997 when Oregon's law went into effect allowing adults with a terminal disease to obtain lethal doses of drugs from their physician, only 171 patients with a terminal disease have taken the medication and died. In 2003, 67 prescriptions for lethal medication were written with 42 deaths secondary to physician-assisted suicide being recorded.

While these numbers are up from 24 requests and 16 deaths in 1998, the numbers remain low and suggest that patients with terminal illnesses are not flocking to doctors for lethal medication to end their lives. One factor keeping the numbers small has been that the law excludes any non-Oregon resident from receiving lethal medication from a physician.

Another fact that has surprised me is that patients who are requesting lethal medication from their doctors are not depressed or in fear of pain, but rather determined to maintain a sense of control and autonomy over the end of their lives.

It has been reported that only one in five patients list fear of uncontrollable pain as a reason for making a request for lethal medication which may represent an improvement in pain management by physicians in Oregon over the past few years.

Perhaps the controversy surrounding physician-assisted suicide has been instrumental in educating doctors on the importance of adequate pain management, as well as a desire to actually make patients more comfortable during the process of dying.

A concern by opponents of physician-assisted suicide has been that patients might feel pressured to end their lives so as to minimize medical debts which could burden their families and, therefore, they would be more likely to request and take lethal drugs.

Surveys in Oregon, however, have found that of patients requesting lethal doses of medication because of not wanting to be a burden to their family, only 2% stated that their concern was one of being a financial burden.

Fear that the Death with Dignity law would lead to forced euthanasia has so far also been dispelled. The state has not reported any evidence that euthanasia has been practiced, nor have the medical or lay communities reported any scandal.

It seems that those opposed to physician-assisted suicide have, for the most part, been reassured that the process is working reasonably well. This may stem from the fact that the legislators, who drafted the law, wrote it to gain support from the vast majority of Oregon citizens, as well as to have sufficient safeguards against abuse. So far they have succeeded.

The framers of the Death with Dignity law were wise to make it difficult to participate in physician-assisted suicide. Patients are required by law to make two verbal and one written request to a doctor over a 15 day waiting period before being eligible for the medication, and in addition, two doctors have to agree that the patient has a terminal illness, has less than 6 months to live, and is mentally competent to make such a request. In other words, it is not easy to obtain lethal doses of drugs to end one's life in Oregon.

One positive aspect of Oregon's law is that for the first time hospices have begun working with groups involved with physician-assisted suicide. Initially being opposed to the law, hospices have learned that 50% of those rejecting hospice services did so because they believed they were "condescending or arrogant."

In response to these surveys, hospices became responsive and supportive to those patients indicating a desire to participate in physician-assisted suicide. As a result, 75% of patients who have chosen to die as a result of physician-assisted suicide have simultaneously been enrolled in a hospice program.

Perhaps because public education on end of life issues, brought about by the passage of this law, Oregon has become a leader in what is called palliative care. Palliative care involves attempts to relieve pain and other unpleasant symptoms while improving the quality of everyday life for patients dying of a terminal illness. Unlike hospice care, it also involves active treatment of the patient's disease regardless of the prognosis.

Citizens of Oregon with terminal illnesses can utilize the benefits of hospice and palliative care, death at home, as well as the use of physician-assisted suicide. Each of these can bring comfort and control to the death and dying process. Many are claiming that a good death rather than a bad death is now more possible in Oregon than in any other state.

Despite all the positive aspects of what is happening in Oregon, I still worry that legalizing physician-assisted suicide will change the way our society thinks about suicide. It may also change how doctors view life and their role in protecting it.

A physician's duty is to protect life and aid us as we reach death. That aid should be one of comfort, pain relief and assurance that in reaching our final destination, we will maintain our dignity as well our autonomy.

Supreme Court Justice Rehnquist stated what I believe to be true, "Assisted suicide goes counter to American history, traditions, laws and moral values. It is fundamentally incompatible with physicians' role as healer."

Physician-assisted suicide is a complex and emotional medical issue. Despite the fact that three-fourths of Americans support the right to take their lives with the help of their doctor, I believe physicians should deal with the sick and dying in a way that shows compassion and concern without stepping over the line by helping patients kill themselves.

Although Oregon has shown us that physician-assisted suicide can be done in such a manner as to avoid many of the concerns that have been raised, I am not so sure that this would be true for our entire nation.

• • •

MARIJUANA AS MEDICINE

He was my colleague and friend. He was a creative, sensitive, caring and inspiring teacher who was admired, respected and loved by his family, friends, students and patients. He was also dying of cancer.

He knew he was dying and accepted his fate with grace and dignity. What he was not accepting or tolerating well, however, were the terrible side effects of chemotherapy.

Unable to tolerate food because of unrelenting and severe nausea and vomiting, my friend was slowly losing weight and wasting away, his strength taken from the very medication he was taking to prolong his life. Nothing seemed to work. Every possible treatment for nausea and vomiting failed to bring relief and comfort or his appetite back.

If something did not happen soon, the chemotherapy would have to be stopped and any chance for an extended period of remission would probably end. But something did happen. My friend told me about it one beautiful fall day while I sat with him on his porch overlooking the green hills of Tennessee.

My friend had smoked marijuana. Having never smoked or used illegal substances, he was at first reluctant to try the carefully rolled cigarette handed to him. However, he was desperate and sick of being sick, so he agreed to give it a try.

What he found surprised him. The marijuana reduced his nausea, stimulated his appetite and generally elevated his mood. In addition, some of the dull pain caused by the cancer was lessened.

Today, the controversy of whether to legalize marijuana for certain medical conditions continues to be debated by the medical community and society. While polls indicate that a majority of Americans are in favor of legalizing marijuana for medical indications, our politicians are not in agreement.

Although politicians maintain a strong desire to keep marijuana illegal, even for patients who could benefit from its use, surveys show that many oncologists routinely recommend marijuana to their patients to treat the terrible nausea brought on by chemotherapy.

A Harvard study of 2,000 oncologists reported that 44% have, in the past, recommended marijuana to their patients who were undergoing chemotherapy. Many physicians have also noted that marijuana helps combat the wasting syndrome that occurs in many patients with AIDS and cancer.

In addition to these ailments, marijuana is occasionally the only drug that sufficiently lowers ocular pressure in patients with glaucoma and eases spastic episodes in sufferers of multiple sclerosis.

While the basic ingredient of marijuana — THC — is legally available in the form of a synthetic pill called Marinol and only costs several dollars a pill, most patients state that it doesn't have the same beneficial effect. The medical community needs to be able to assist sick individuals in their efforts to live a reasonably comfortable life until the inevitability of death occurs.

Hopefully, our government will someday allow physicians to prescribe marijuana to certain patients. Physicians are well-schooled in prescribing controlled substances such as morphine and Demerol. There is no reason why they could not do the same with marijuana.

・・・

FREE NEEDLES

My patient was stunned. "How could I be HIV positive?" she asked. She had been in a monogamous relationship for five years, did not use illegal drugs and never had a blood transfusion. I couldn't answer her.

I only knew that her prenatal tests had revealed her to be infected with the AIDS virus, and unless we treated her aggressively during pregnancy, her unborn child had a significant chance of being infected as well.

Several weeks later she returned to my office with the answer. Her boyfriend admitted that he used intravenous heroin, shared needles with friends, and was also HIV positive. My patient's world collapsed around her; she was devastated.

What is especially sad about this story is that it could have been so easily prevented.

One of the most effective and inexpensive methods of preventing the spread of HIV is a needle exchange program. Because intravenous drug addicts cannot buy new syringes without a prescription, syringes are used over and over by multiple addicts, thus spreading the AIDS virus from one person to another. These infected intravenous drug users then spread the disease through heterosexual contact to their partners and, if female, they in turn can spread the virus to their unborn child.

The Center for Disease Control claims that this method of spread now accounts for over a third of all new HIV cases each year. A needle exchange program seeks to change this pattern by giving free sterile syringes to drug addicts.

Beginning in Boston many years ago, there are now over one hundred needle exchange programs in over 71 cities, collecting and distributing approximately ten million syringes each year. But this is not enough to stem the tide. Unfortunately, current law prohibits federal funds for free clean needle programs.

According to some in Congress, the ban might be lifted if it could be proven that needle exchange programs do not lead to an increase in drug use, which is difficult to prove. What is much easier to prove, however, and has been proven, is that needle exchange programs decrease HIV spread.

In 1997, the Department of Health and Human Services declared that needle exchange programs did retard HIV transmission.

In addition, a 1995 National Academy of Sciences National Research Council report found that needle exchange programs prevent spread of HIV, while not increasing the use of illicit drugs. One reason these programs work is they also offer counseling and drug treatment referrals to those receiving new syringe and needles.

Many prestigious organizations are in support of needle exchange programs, including the American Medical Association, the American Bar Association, the Association of State and Territorial Health Officials, the CDC, the US Conference of Mayors, and the American Public Health Association. So why the controversy?

It mainly lies with the American people! Polls show that Americans generally oppose needle exchange programs. One survey revealed 62% in opposition to such exchange programs, with 60% of the people supporting drug abstinence and drug rehabilitation as a better way to stop the spread of AIDS.

More troubling is that these surveys also reveal a belief that federal government's support of needle exchange programs represents government endorsement of illegal drug use.

It's too bad Americans feel this way. It has been estimated that if America had initiated a widely promoted needle exchange program in 1987, we could have prevented as many as 10,000 HIV infections by 1995. Besides lives spared, think about the money that could have also been saved.

Once again public health is another name for political health and it is my innocent pregnant patient and her unborn child who suffer the consequences.

• • •

THE MYSTERY AND PAIN OF SUICIDE

Not only was he the most handsome of our young teenage group of boys, Pat was a great athlete, very smart, extremely popular and dated the prettiest girl I had ever seen. In truth, I was quite envious of him as I attempted to traverse those pimple-filled insecure high school years back in the 1950s. Pat seemed to have it all. Or so I thought!

When he killed himself during our senior year in high school, I was stunned and bewildered. Why would someone with so much to live for kill himself?

We have all known or heard of others who have committed suicide. Over the years I have tried to understand why, but each time I heard of another appearingly senseless suicide the same lack of understanding surfaced.

The last few years, however, I have come to understand at least one of the reasons someone might commit suicide. Despite his outside demeanor, my high school friend was probably depressed. Studies reveal that one half of manic depressive individuals will attempt suicide, and one out of five with significant depression will also make that same attempt.

Kay Jamison's writing in her book about suicide, *Night Falls Fast,* states that mental disorders may have their origin in organic, as well as social causes. She hypothesizes that fetal exposure to alcohol or cocaine, lack of motherly attention in early childhood, or even improper diet may lead to later mood disorders that then may result in suicide.

In addition, Jamison claims that genetic factors probably also play an important role in predisposing an individual to mental disease, as well as such personality traits as impulsiveness, aggression and violence, which in turn may also lead to suicide.

Whatever the underlying factors that lead to suicide, there is general agreement that suicide is a huge public health problem, as well as a personal tragedy. Jamison reports that every 17 minutes someone in the United States commits suicide.

Suicide ranks third in causes of young people's deaths and second for college students. More men under the age of 35 die of suicide than of AIDS. In addition to the actual death from suicide, 500,000 Americans each year attempt suicide.

What is quite troubling is that the rate of suicide is alarmingly doubling among children ages 10 through 14 just in the last 20 years. The big question, of course, is what our society can do about this chronic problem.

Jamison is not happy with the media which she believes attempts to separate suicide from mental illness, as well as putting suicidal ideas into its audience's minds (she reminds us that suicide is "contagious" as seen in localized suicidal epidemics). She is equally unhappy with our current medical care system which does not administer appropriate coverage or treatment to the mentally ill.

Studies reveal that up to 90% of suicidal teenagers suffer from some form of psychological illness and that their suicide is usually not an impulsive act.

However, while Jamison has a point, teenage depression can be very difficult to recognize. A study of high school counselors found that two out of every three professional counselors admitted that they could not spot the warning signs of a potential suicidal student!

What I have found out about suicide can be best summed up by Jamison's telling of her own suicidal attempt. "No amount of love from or for other people could help. No advantage of a caring family and fabulous job was enough to overcome the pain and hopelessness I felt; no passionate or romantic love, however strong, could make a difference. Nothing alive and warm could make its way in through my carapace. I knew my life could be a shambles and I believed that my family, friends and patients would be better off without me. There wasn't much of me left anymore. Anyway, I thought my death would free up the wasted energies and well-meant efforts that were being wasted in my behalf."

Perhaps family and friends left behind can at least rid themselves of some of the guilt by understanding the absolute loss of hope with a mixture of incredible psychic pain that occurs in those who commit suicide.

Where our kids are concerned I suppose all we can try to do is talk to them and let them know that many teenagers get depressed and that if they do, they don't need to suffer ... there is medical treatment.

I just wish my friend, Pat, had known this.

• • •

INSANITY OR MURDER: POSTPARTUM DEPRESSION

If ever there was a good argument for an insanity defense, it was the case of Andrea Pia Yates. On June 20, 2001 37-year-old Andrea Yates of Clear Lake, Texas, drowned her 5 children (Noah 7, John 5, Paul 3, Luke 2 and Mary 6 months) in a bathtub and faced the death penalty for her actions.

Defense attorneys for Ms. Yates claimed that Andrea suffered from postpartum psychosis when she drowned her children and that she should not have been tried as a mentally competent adult. I totally agree.

Having practiced Obstetrics for 35 years, I have seen postpartum depression, as well as a few cases of postpartum psychosis up close. After reading many of the details of the Yates case, I was convinced that she should have been admitted to a psychiatric hospital, treated with appropriate anti-psychotic medication and extensively counseled for a very long time, perhaps her entire life. This did not happen.

A jury of 11 women and one man found Andrea mentally competent to stand trial on capital murder charges and later a jury found her guilty of first degree murder and sentenced Andrea to life in prison. Fortunately, in early January 2005, an appeals court in Houston ruled that a prosecution expert's false testimony required a retrial.

For reasons that are not well understood, approximately 15% of women having delivered a baby will develop clinical depression. While there are associated risk factors such as low self-esteem, family history of depression, single marital status, medically indigent and a previous bout of postpartum depression (50-100% recurrence rate), some women develop postpartum depression without any type of warning.

Most clinicians now believe that postpartum depression is a biomolecular problem which often requires antidepressant medication and careful follow-up with medical personnel, an approach which usually results in complete cure.

However, in a few cases (1 in 1000) a much more serious ailment of clinical psychosis becomes apparent. This diagnosis can be made when suicidal thoughts or attempts occur, or if the patient has delusional thoughts. Clearly, Andrea Yates fell into that category.

Andrea Yates did not manifest symptoms of depression until six months after the birth of her fourth child, Luke, when she attempted to kill herself with her father's Alzheimer's prescription medication. Following this first suicidal attempt, Andrea was hospitalized for a week, treated with antidepressant medication and then released, in part, because of insurance problems. Physicians believed that while she was still depressed, she was no longer suicidal. Obviously they were wrong.

A few weeks later, having stopped taking her medication, Andrea Yates began hearing voices and having destructive visions. Her husband, Russell Yates, readmitted Andrea to the hospital when he found his wife holding a knife to her neck, threatening to kill herself. This time she spent 19 days in the hospital and was noted to improve as she underwent group therapy and, more importantly, was placed on an effective anti-psychotic medication.

Then came the birth of Andrea Yates's fifth child, Mary, and with it another bout of severe postpartum psychosis. This psychosis, manifested by such symptoms as catatonia and scratching her head bald, required four voluntary admissions to a psychiatric hospital.

On the day of her last discharge from the hospital, May 14, records indicate that Andrea was depressed and still having suicidal thoughts. She drowned her five children 37 days later.

What caused Andrea Yates to develop postpartum psychosis will probably never be known. We are, however, told some interesting facts that could help explain some of the reasons she became so sick.

Andrea's father, two brothers and a sister have a history of mental illness. Andrea had thoughts of hurting her child as early as the birth of her first son, Noah, and then developed a full blown case of depression after the birth of her fourth child. After she improved with treatment she was then subjected to yet another pregnancy.

In addition, Andrea was under considerable stress. Along with having to care for her children in a converted Greyhound bus, as well as having to care for her ailing father, Andrea home-schooled her kids and had no more than two hours a week of free time just for herself.

With a strong family history, a previous bout of severe postpartum psychosis, which is associated with a 5% incidence of infanticide, as well as living under enormous stress as a homemaker, mother and wife, can there be any doubt that Andrea Yates drowned her children because of insanity?

Most parents would, without hesitation, sacrifice their lives to save their children if the need arose. Andrea Yates did the unthinkable when she drowned her five children on June 20. But she did not do it because she wanted a better life.

She had been pleading for help and her cries went unanswered. She killed her children because she was mentally ill and could not help herself. If that is not insanity, I do not know what is.

・・・

IT'S IN YOUR HEAD

It has been over 40 years since I began my formal training as a first year medical student at Vanderbilt University and I marvel how much in medicine has changed. While much can be said about the technical advances in every specialty, I am particularly impressed with the changes in our thinking about certain illnesses that were once labeled as "mental."

I remember, for example, being taught as a young student that many psychotic and neurotic illnesses were, to a large degree, environmentally caused. How you related to your mother or father were important factors to consider in treating many mental problems.

Many other problems were also believed to be in our patient's head and not a medical disorder; depression could be overcome with a good pep talk, behavioral disorders with punishment or reward, and severe unrelenting vomiting in pregnancy with counseling to treat the possibility that the patient was ambivalent about her pregnancy.

Another teaching of the early 1960s was that severe menstrual cramps, unresponsive to conventional therapy, were possibly caused in part or affected by a woman's denial of her femininity.

I can remember sending all too many women with such problems to psychiatrists for treatment, hoping that through counseling, their pain would either lessen or be more manageable.

As we now know, it was the wrong therapy. No one improved and the severe menstrual cramps continued. It was 1972 when a patient with severe menstrual cramps was sent to me in the hopes that we might know of some new breakthrough in the treatment of this disorder called dysmenorrhea.

The patient was in her thirties, pleasant and well-educated. She was married, childless and had been through every type of treatment imaginable including pain medication, hormones and multiple surgical procedures. She had also undergone a three month trial of psychotherapy by a psychiatrist in town.

Nothing worked. Each month, she was bedridden for approximately three days in excruciating pain requiring narcotics and resulting in loss of work, self-esteem and productivity at home. Nothing was left except a total hysterectomy which, while the ultimate cure, would also result in her remaining childless forever — something she was not ready to consider.

The first time I met with her, she explained to me that the medical profession labeled her problem as one that might be in her head, but she knew better. Why couldn't physicians understand this problem and come up with a cure?

I searched the literature for new clues and talked to colleagues working on this problem all over the country. I learned of a very exciting discovery of a naturally occurring substance called prostaglandin that scientists had isolated and found in higher than normal concentrations in the uterus of a woman with dysmenorrhea. The worse the dysmenorrhea, the higher the levels of this compound.

Prostaglandin causes the uterus to contract and is one of the most potent uterine contractile substances known. It was determined that this new hormone could be prevented from reaching high levels by using a very strong aspirin-like drug called Indocin.

At the time, Indocin was used mainly for patients with arthritis. I discussed this new information with my patient and she agreed to try it. We started her on Indocin before her severe menstrual cramps began and her next menses was totally painless. She was ecstatic and had tears of joy as she told me of her cure.

This patient led me and her referring doctor to study 30 other patients with similar outcomes which resulted in our publishing our findings in the *Journal of Reproductive Medicine* in 1975.

Today, after years of research, we know of many medicines such as Indocin (like Ibuprofin) that have a profound effect on curing dysmenorrhea, a disorder once thought only to be in a woman's head.

There are numerous other examples which have changed our entire thinking of illness. Now, many psychotic and neurotic diseases are being treated with compounds directly affecting various chemical and electrical reactions in the brain.

Just as diabetes is a disease which requires the replacement of insulin to the body because of a failure of the pancreatic gland to secrete the proper amount of insulin, so are many mental illnesses the result of such chemical alterations and not merely a result of how we were raised at home.

What this teaches us is that many "illnesses" the medical profession often label as "in our head," like premenstrual syndrome, chronic fatigue syndrome, pain in various parts of the body, behavioral disorders, or even postpartum depression, are only waiting for a scientific breakthrough to understand what is really going on.

• • •

SEXUAL INFORMATION

The year was 1969 and I was 29-years-old. Having completed my training in obstetrics and gynecology, I felt adept at taking care of all aspects of pregnancy as well as being able to perform routine and complicated reproductive operations and procedures.

Yet, when a patient asked if I could help her with a sexual problem she was having, I was ill-equipped.

You see, no one throughout my medical school or residency program had ever brought up the subject of sexual dysfunction. This extremely important aspect of human behavior was simply not included in the curriculum. Therefore, I sought the help and advice of my teachers. Surely they knew how I could help my patient. Sadly, they only shrugged their shoulders and offered little or no help.

I was amazed. How could the medical profession ignore this vital human function in the education of its students?

I told my anxious patient that I needed to look into the subject. I promised I would do my best to educate myself about her problem so I could give her proper professional advice.

Unfortunately, there was little material to help me. Books, lay and professional, were interesting but not of the same caliber that I had come to expect from medical textbooks that were usually so helpful in educating me on a variety of other medical problems.

Although too late for my patient, eventually I did make progress. I participated in a week long Sexual Attitude Reassessment Workshop in Minneapolis which I found to be quite helpful.

Combined with being a regular facilitator at Sexual Attitude Reassessment weekends in Nashville and running a Sexual Dysfunction Clinic at our hospital, I slowly found myself becoming more proficient in helping women with their sexual dysfunction complaints. I also started teaching medical students and residents on this immensely important subject.

Because of my interest in the field of sexual counseling I was not surprised to read a report on sexual dysfunction in the United States published in the *Journal of the American Medical Association.*

A survey of over 1400 men and 1700 women between 18 and 59 years of age found that 43% of women and 31% of men complained of sexual dysfunction. Sexual dysfunction was identified as a lack of desire, arousal problems, and inability to achieve orgasm, anxiety about sexual performance, premature ejaculation, and painful or unpleasurable intercourse.

The media made much of this survey. Newspaper headlines, such as "Study Dispels Nation's Glorified Myth of Sex" were common throughout the country. Yet health care professionals who deal with sexual dysfunction were not surprised by the findings of the survey.

While television, movies and magazines portray a sex-crazed society, Americans are anything but. Study co-author, Raymond C. Rosen, stated that all too often a person's perception of what their sex lives should be are dictated by magazines, which often give the impression that everyone else is having incredible sex all the time. The fact is that while often the interest may be there the performance is not.

Unfortunately, the medical profession is still woefully undereducated on how to deal with problems concerning sexual dysfunction. We are doing a better job in this regard, however, we still have a long way to go.

While it is true that erectile dysfunction medications have come to the rescue of many men, it is also clear that we have done very little in this country to help women with problems of achieving orgasm or painful and unpleasurable sex. We must address this issue of sexual dysfunction and give aid and comfort to those who wish to be helped.

Now that we have better information on the frequency of sexual dysfunction, it is up to the medical profession to make sure that physicians and patients do not have to go through the same kind of experience my patient and I had many years ago.

• • •

HEART OF A WOMAN

"I am having chest pain" the 28-year-old female patient told the nurse as she was being admitted to the Vanderbilt Emergency Room. "When did the chest pain start?" the nurse asked as she finished taking this new patient's blood pressure, pulse and temperature. "Early this morning I woke up with my chest hurting and feeling weak. By the way, I am 12 weeks pregnant." The nurse finished her preliminary work, filling out the necessary forms and left the exam room to find the doctor on-call.

"It is probably indigestion" the emergency room physician explained. "I doubt it is anything serious, but just to be on the safe side, I would like you to have an electrocardiogram. If that is normal, I believe we can send you home with antacids."

Minutes later, upon reviewing the electrocardiogram, the emergency room doctor realized his patient was not suffering from indigestion. She was having a heart attack!

Despite the fact that she was only 28-years-old, did not smoke, and had no family history of heart disease, this wise, careful, and thorough ER doctor knew that women, just like men, can suffer from coronary heart disease, and therefore, ordered an electrocardiogram ... just to be sure.

More than likely he saved her life. Within hours, the patient had undergone cardiac catheterization, as well as treatment with a clot-busting drug given directly into the coronary artery and was now feeling great.

Several months later, and with no further problems, the patient delivered a healthy child in our Labor and Delivery Suite, just three floors above the emergency room where she had initially sought medical care for chest pain.

Cardiovascular disease, which includes heart attacks and strokes, is the leading cause of death in women in the United States. Records indicate that over 40% of all deaths of women in this country are caused by cardiovascular disease, and not all of these deaths are in older women. Many heart attack patients are women under the age of 50.

The good news concerning cardiovascular disease in women is twofold. One is that the medical profession is now more aware that women can suffer from coronary heart disease. Therefore, they are more likely to look for undiagnosed heart problems in women of all ages who present with complaints consistent with heart disease. Secondly, there is evidence that coronary heart disease in women is on the decline.

A survey published in the *New England Journal of Medicine* revealed that among approximately 86,000 nurses followed from 1980 to 1994, the incidence of coronary heart disease dropped by 31%. Criticized for not studying heart disease in women, the medical profession began The Nurse's Health Study in 1976.

The study enrolled over 120,000 female nurses between the ages of 30 and 55 who had agreed to a long-term study of their medical history and lifestyle habits. Analyzing the data collected on a significant portion of this group, the authors of this report found that smoking declined by 41% and diet was significantly improved. These factors helped explained the decline in the rate of heart disease.

That bit of good news, however, is tempered somewhat by the fact that during this same time interval, the number of women who were considered overweight increased by 38%, thereby slowing the overall decline of coronary heart disease.

The authors concluded that "the increase of weight among women from 1980 to 1994, despite other improvements in lifestyle variables, is disappointing and undoubtedly mirrors trends among men and children as well."

Over the past ten years this increase in obesity has also been associated with an increase in the incidence of diabetes mellitus in the United States. Diabetes significantly increases the incidence and severity of heart disease, and, therefore, adds to the burden of women trying to stay healthy.

In other words, the fact we are becoming more and more overweight in this country is slowing the decline in heart disease despite all the other good things that we are doing. Coronary heart disease is a complex problem that is a result of a number of genetic and environmental factors.

Nonetheless, it is crucial for all of us to adhere to a healthy lifestyle, which includes exercising, eating a healthy diet, watching our blood pressure and cholesterol levels, stop smoking and keeping our weight down by consuming less calories.

While these lifestyle changes can have a dramatic effect on heart disease, it is still critical that doctors and nurses be alert to the typical signs and symptoms of heart disease, even in a 28-year-old pregnant woman.

. . .

GET OFF THE COUCH

The Institute of Medicine is claiming Americans need to exercise at least an hour a day to maintain good health (which is twice as much as has been previously recommended). I couldn't help but think, "Are they kidding?"

For the past 35 years, I have been encouraging my patients, many who were postpartum, to begin an exercise program in an effort to help lose weight and prevent heart disease. However, I have only been moderately successful, in part due to the fact that many Americans either have difficulty finding the time it takes to exercise or simply have no interest in exercising.

Based on a 1995 recommendation by the Center for Disease Control and the American College of Sports Medicine, as well as a 1996 recommendation by the United States Surgeon General, it was advised that 30 minutes of moderately intense physical activity each day of the week should be initiated to attain and maintain good health. I suggested to my patients that brisk walking for 30 minutes each day was recommended and required to reduce the risk of cardiac problems as well as to stabilize weight.

But following this recommendation was difficult for many of my patients who claim that they have considerable trouble finding 30 minutes each day to exercise. Many people live hectic, full lives with very little spare time available for prolonged exercising.

Waking at 6 a.m. to get a family ready for school and work, followed by a sprint to the grocery store, fixing dinner, getting children through homework, bathed and into bed, leaves many Americans much too tired to participate in exercise.

Imagine the problem Americans will have with the Institute of Medicine's recommendation that they should exercise an hour a day!

The Institute of Medicine's 21 experts who wrote the 1000 page report were concerned about the huge number of overweight Americans and made sweeping recommendations concerning diet and exercise. The panel of experts advised that both adults and children spend at least one hour daily in moderately intense physical activities such as swimming, bicycling, jogging or brisk walking.

Fortunately, not everyone is in agreement with this new recommendation. Some scientists are claiming that given the fact that 60% of Americans are couch potatoes and do no exercising whatsoever, and the other 40% struggle to find time each day to perform some form of physical exertion, this recommendation is impractical. I would add that it is also counterproductive in helping convince Americans to begin an exercise program or continue the one they are currently doing.

Why should you continue walking 30 minutes a day if there is no benefit? And, if you know you will never be able to find the required hour a day for exercising, why exercise at all?

In 2002 the *New England Journal of Medicine* addressed this issue. Examining the effects of physical activity on over 70,000 women between the ages of 50 and 79 years, the authors concluded that women who spent between 45 minutes and seven hours a week walking had 3.6 to 7.8 fewer heart attacks for every 1000 participants during the three years of the study.

In addition, the study revealed that there was a similar reduction in heart attacks with either walking or more vigorous activity, although the study also demonstrated that those women who exercised the most had a higher health benefit with a gradual reduction of benefits as time spent exercising decreased.

The bottom line, however, was that the study found that those women who walked briskly for 30 minutes a day, five days a week had 30% less heart attacks than those women who were not as active.

There is also similar convincing data in studies involving men. That should be good news for those individuals who are exercising at that level and should be encouraging to those who are considering starting an exercise program.

Large numbers of studies have concluded that exercise is beneficial for good health. How much, how long and what type of exercise, however, has not been totally answered.

While the study of women and exercise suggests that an hour a day of moderately intense exercise (mild shortness of breath) is optimal, there still is considerable benefit from less time spent exercising.

I have been successful in convincing some of my patients on the importance of finding 30 minutes early in the morning or before dinner to briskly walk around the neighborhood. However, finding an hour would not be an easy task.

Before we attempt to convince Americans that they should exercise an hour a day, perhaps we should first encourage them to exercise thirty minutes, which would be beneficial to their overall physical and mental health and help keep body weight down.

Current data indicate that only 25% of Americans meet national guidelines for 30 minutes of brisk walking or its equivalent 5 days a week. We must improve this figure if we are going to reduce heart disease as well as interrupt the continuing increase of obesity being observed in this country.

There is no easy formula for being in good physical health. Reducing caloric intake, taking preventive health measures and getting off the couch to walk briskly 30 minutes each day is a very good start. As the Nike ad says, "Just do it."

• • •

THE BIBLE AND YOUR HEALTH

While I do not recommend that doctors stop reading medical books and journals in search of information to help Americans live healthy lives, I do recommend obtaining additional information from another source ... the Bible.

Two examples are worth telling. Judges 13:4 tells of an angel telling Manoah's wife that she was soon to conceive a son (who would be called Sampson) and that once pregnant, she should, "... drink no wine nor strong drink." This warning to not drink alcohol when pregnant surely is the first time in history that we learn of potential adverse side effects of alcohol on the fetus.

It took until 1968 before the medical literature would acknowledge and describe distinct fetal abnormalities, which is now called fetal alcohol syndrome. While we first learned of this from the Bible, we now know that excessive alcohol intake during pregnancy can cause miscarriage, improper fetal growth of body and brain, facial and heart abnormalities, mental retardation, developmental delay, hyperactivity and attention deficit syndrome.

The second example comes from Exodus 20:8-11. It is here that the Lord tells us to, "Remember the Sabbath day, to keep it holy. Six days shalt thou labor and do all thy work; but the seventh day is a Sabbath unto the Lord thy God, in it thou shalt not do any manner of work." This biblical commandment is especially important for Americans to heed in today's stressed and hectic way of life.

American workers are stressed out and this stress is affecting health. Surveys indicate that over 60% of American workers claim their work has increased in the past six months and that over half claim their work leaves them "overworked and overwhelmed."

Experts claim that stress levels at work are much higher today than they were just a few years ago. According to the National Opinion Research Center at the University of Chicago, over 30% of American workers claim that they are "always" or "often" under stress at work.

Americans are working harder today than they ever have, putting in over 1,800 hours on the job each year, a figure that is 350 hours more than in Germany and slightly more than in Japan. In addition, because of advanced technology, workers are really never off the job. With cell phones and e-mail, which now can be handheld and portable, there is no good way to avoid being available to the needs of a job 24 hours a day, 7 days a week. White-collar workers, who tend to take their work home, are particularly hit the hardest.

This environment is literally making many of us sick. Medical research has shown that stress is related to acute and chronic illness and has the potential to kill.

Heart attacks, strokes, depression, anxiety, gastro-intestinal problems and loss of immunity to illnesses are but a few of the side effects of being overly stressed. Chronic stress can also lead to sleep deprivation, as well as overeating which then can lead to obesity and diabetes.

Reduction of stress has been shown to reduce many of these problems and result in a significant improvement of health. In addition, it could also reduce the enormous amount of money lost by business because of additional health care cost and missed work for stressed workers. It has been estimated that workplace stress costs our country over $300 billions each year!

Studies also show that when stress in the workplace increases, such as when downsizing occurs or with large-scale expansions and reorganizations, the risk of death secondary to heart attack, increase in blood pressure and cholesterol levels, all increased significantly. Employees are turning to antidepressant and anti-anxiety medication to cope with this increased stress during the workweek.

Perhaps Americans should consider following the fourth commandment. Because workers are overworked and stressed during the week, it makes sense that what is needed is a real day of rest, as the Bible prescribes.

That rest could be obtained by turning off cell phones, beepers and computers, letting answering machines take messages to be retrieved later, taking time for reflection on walks or at a house of worship, or just being at home with family and friends.

Our brain and body need downtime. Without this downtime, we continue to run the risk of disease and early death. In addition to not smoking, exercising, eating properly, getting sufficient sleep, and practicing preventive medicine, we desperately need a real day of rest each and every week. That commandment written thousands of years ago has never been as important as it is today.

• • •

TOO MANY CHOICES

A few years ago it was reported that there had been a threefold increase in clinical depression in this country over the past 25 years and a tenfold increase since the beginning of the 20th century.

In addition, over the past 30 years, the proportion of Americans describing themselves as "happy" has declined. With all the advances in living that we have experienced over the past 25-100 years, I can't help but wonder what might lie at the root of all this depression and unhappiness?

It seems that while our living conditions have improved, we have become more depressed and less happy. Life expectancy has increased from 47 at the beginning of the 20th century to 77 years today.

We have stamped out many common diseases, improved survival rates of patients with cancer, lowered the incidence of heart disease, stroke, and cancer, lowered child poverty rates, increased the purchasing power of the average American, reduced smog in our cities, increased the number of young adults who have graduated from college, and significantly lowered traffic fatalities, just to name a few facts that reveal an improvement of life in America.

Yes, we still have many serious problems facing us, but you have to ask yourself, if life is so much better today, why do we seem so depressed, anxious, restless and frustrated?

Perhaps the answer to this question has something to do with the fact that Americans have too many choices! That is what Barry Schwartz, a psychology professor at Swarthmore College and author of *The Paradox of Choice: Why More is Less* believes. I think he may be onto something.

Americans are bombarded with choices everywhere they turn. Just go into a local drug store and attempt to purchase toothpaste. I used to just buy toothpaste, but the other day as I stood in front of the shelf with the many choices in front of me, I felt confused and frustrated. There are 40 types to pick from so how do I know which one was best for me?

It does not stop there. With over 80 kinds of painkillers, 360 types of shampoo and hair conditioners, dozens of different kinds of breads, chips, colas and cereals, just going out for medications or food can be daunting.

Multiples of choices are everywhere we look. Want to choose: the best and cheapest telephone service, a mobile phone or camera, the best car, TV, pair of shoes or item on a dinner menu, a retirement or health insurance plan, purchasing a mattress, a computer that best meets your needs, the best college to go to, as well as the best job to take after college, a person to date or marry?

As Schwartz points out, more choice has the tendency to lead to a decline in satisfaction, and that too many choices can result in paralysis, not liberation. He sites a few examples that prove his point. As the choices for jam or chocolates increases for shoppers, the more likely it is that the shopper will leave the grocery store without purchasing the item. In fact, shoppers are ten times more likely to buy jam when six different types are available as when there are 24 on the shelf.

More to the point, Schwartz describes a study that noted that as the number of job possibilities available to graduating college students increases, satisfaction with the job search decreases.

Those students searching for the very best job in this environment of many choices, report less satisfied with their eventual choice and also were found to be more anxious, pessimistic, disappointed, frustrated and depressed.

Even with the task of choosing a 401k retirement plan, the more choices employees are given, the more they opt not to choose any.

Patients who are undergoing treatment for cancer are often frustrated with the many choices the health care system asks them to make. Most want to let the doctor make the choices. They do not want to make life and death decisions, they do not want that kind of responsibility. I cannot tell you how many times I have been asked, "what would you do, Doctor?"

Too many choices have the potential to create a feeling of frustration and anxiety, and these choices place an enormous burden on individuals who have to do the homework in order to make the best choice. And often, when the choice is finally made, there is a lingering doubt that the right choice was made (which then has the potential to create feelings of missed opportunities and regret).

As if all this were not bad enough, Schwartz points out that "an abundance of options raises people's expectation about how good the option they have chosen will be, and that increased choices force people to take personal responsibility for all choices that turn out to be less than perfect." What a huge responsibility!

Put in other words, fewer choices can actually lead to a sense of more freedom, less anxiety and frustration and perhaps even less depression. This may not be a prescription for all that ails Americans, but it sure would help me select a toothpaste.

I wish I could offer a solution for the problem of having too many choices in our society. There were, however, so many solutions to choose from, that I simply could not make up my mind which one to recommend.

• • •

CAN WE KNOW TOO MUCH

During a philosophical discussion on death and dying a few years ago, the question was raised whether any of us would want to know when we were going to die. A friend of mine responded by saying he did not want to know when he was going to die, but did want to know where. When queried as to why, he stated that if he knew where he was going to die, he would never go there.

We all laughed at our friend's sense of humor, yet that discussion raised an important sense of awareness for me. Do any of us really want to know when or even how we are going to die? I believe most would not.

Yet, we have entered an era in medical history when, with genetic testing, we are being told many facts concerning our genetic make-up. We are given information that is highly predictive of many diseases, such as cancer and heart disease, and may pinpoint with some accuracy when as well as how we are probably going to die.

Huntington disease serves as a useful model and example of this new evolving concept of using genetic information to help manage our health. Huntington disease affects about 25,000 Americans and is a severe neurological disease which occurs at an individual's mid-life ultimately leading to death after ten to 15 years of uncontrollable psychological deterioration and dementia.

Unfortunately, patients with Huntington disease pass their genetic defect to 50% of their children. Thus, children of those affected know that they have a 50/50 chance of having the disease long before the first symptoms appear.

Many offspring of patients with Huntington disease are considering whether they should request available genetic testing to determine if they are going to eventually be afflicted with this disease. Because there is no cure or treatment, individuals at potential risk undergo an incredible emotionally wrenching experience deciding whether or not to be tested.

Would it be better not to know? Or would knowing bring an element of emotional peace?

As it turns out, there is an available answer to this question. A Canadian collaborative study published in *The New England Journal of Medicine* reported that in a group of at-risk individuals for Huntington disease, those who chose to have themselves tested regardless of the outcome, had better psychological health after being tested than those who chose not to be tested.

I believe individuals with a strong family history of other diseases such as breast, colon or ovarian cancer, which also have genetic tests, and are highly predictive of whether an individual will develop cancer, should consider availing themselves to this type of genetic testing. Unlike Huntington's disease, something can be done to prevent these cancers from causing death if detected early.

Some day there will be genetic testing that uncovers a high risk status for heart disease, obesity, alcoholism, psychiatric and personality disorders, Alzheimer's dementia, diabetes, hypertension and perhaps even sexual orientation. How our society will handle this information remains unanswered.

Daily ethical issues are arising from this aspect of predictive genetic testing. While the right to know is well established in American medicine, the right not to know has not been critically evaluated by physicians or patients.

As we learn more about our genetic make-up and are able to predict more and more influencing diseases and conditions, our society should start thinking about what to do with this information.

As better technology leads to advances in genetic testing and we learn more about our genetic make-up, we may one day know when we are going to die. The question we must then ask is no joke. Do we want to go there?

• • •

THE PERFECT CHILD

Over the past 38 years, I have participated in the care of thousands of pregnant women and have attempted to answer the many questions that each patient invariably wants answered.

While these questions are often specific to each patient's pregnancy, one common question usually surfaces at some point in our discussion, "Is my baby OK?" Because it is so difficult for me to define "OK," this question has always been a tough one for me to answer.

At the heart of this question lies a pregnant patient's desire to know if her unborn child will be perfect (normal and healthy), a very reasonable concern. Once again, however, defining perfect is not an easy task.

Most pregnant women do not realize that approximately 2% of the 4 million births each year in this country involve the delivery of a child with a significant congenital defect. That translates to one out of 50 births!

These birth defects include hundreds of different types of anomalies such as spina bifida, heart abnormalities, limb deformities, metabolic disorders and chromosomal abnormalities such as Down syndrome.

When you consider that each of us begins with the union of sperm and egg, which creates one cell and this one cell continuously divides to create the billions of cells that result in a living child, it is truly a miracle that any of us are born, much less that we are born perfect.

It is with this in mind that I explain to patients that each birth is a miracle and that the uniqueness of each of us is what makes us perfect. I also attempt to explain that normal is in the eye of the beholder. The gift of life can be "perfect" even in the presence of serious problems.

In August of 2003, my newly born grandson, Seth, was to help me understand this from a different perspective. Seth was born with Down syndrome.

Down syndrome was first described by Dr. John Langdon Down in 1866 as a condition in which a child is short in stature with mild to moderate mental retardation, as well as often being associated with other physical problems such as heart defects.

The risk of having a child with Down syndrome increases as women age. At 20 years of age, the risk is one in 2,000 births and at 35 it is one in 365. At age 40, the risk of delivering a child with Down syndrome is one in 100.

I have spent my entire career counseling patients on the risk of delivering a child with Down syndrome. But until the birth of Seth, I had never been confronted on a personal level.

My son Tommy and his wife Lisa were expecting twins — a girl and a boy. I vividly remember the excitement as my wife, Julie, and I waited during the delivery and cried with joy as we each held a child in our arms in the recovery room. Marly and Seth were perfect. What dreams and expectations we held for these two precious bundles of joy!

Several hours later, however, we were confronted with the fact that Seth carried a diagnosis of Down syndrome while his sister Marly did not. Our family was filled with emotions, from the high that came with the birth of the twins to a low at learning of Seth's disability and knowing that he would be different with possible lifelong problems.

Later that evening, holding Seth in my arms and gazing into his angelic face, I was overcome with unconditional love for my grandson.

As the tears rolled down my cheek, I understood that despite his diagnosis, to me and those who love him, Seth is a perfect child, to be loved and nurtured, the same as his sister Marly. Our dreams and expectations for him may now be different from those for his sister, yet they are dreams and expectations nonetheless.

To me, Seth is perfect. His smile lights up a room and his laughter brings warmth to all who are near. He loves to cuddle and gaze into the eyes of those who hold him, and he embraces his sister with what can only be described as pure affection and love.

Seth is one of many children who are born with birth defects and complications, yet, like so many others, Seth has embarked on a journey we call life. That life will be filled with challenges for him and his family, yet that is also true of each of us as we embrace life with its ups and downs.

As we enter a world in which more genetic information will be available for us to consider in selecting a perfect child, I hope we have room in our world and hearts for those like Seth who are challenged and different, because challenged and different can still be perfect.

• • •

BIRTH ORDER MATTERS

My second child, Tommy, now 37-years-old, recently asked me a penetrating and somewhat uncomfortable question "Dad, you have written newspaper columns about Todd (my firstborn) and Catherine (my baby), yet you have never written one about me, how come?"

It was true. I had written about Todd leaving home for college, his marriage and the birth of his first child. I had written about Catherine's Bat Mitzvah in Israel, her reaching puberty and my difficulty with telling her about sex, and finally, her leaving home for college. Yet I had never written a column about Tommy.

No awkward response seemed to work for him or for me for that matter, and so I decided to do some research. After all, I love my son Tommy just as much as my two other children. He is a sensitive, compassionate, caring, thought provoking, religious, honest and highly intelligent young man. Surely there was an answer to his question. Why had I not written a column about him?

In an effort to answer that question, I found a book written by Dr. Kevin Leman entitled *The New Birth Order Book*. Leman notes that "it is quite normal for middle children to feel left out, ignored and even insulted."

Leman also adds that being a middle child is very difficult to describe or even generalize in any meaningful way. Yet, the author of this interesting book describes a middle child as one who typically goes off in a different direction than his older brother or sister, and while "any number of lifestyles can appear they all play off the firstborn."

Most of the research on middle children indicates that the second born most likely will be somewhat opposite to their older sibling.

It seems that because the oldest and the youngest get most of the attention, the middle child feels as if they have to do whatever it takes to get some attention. Sometimes that works, oftentimes it does not. Frequently, parental awareness of the needs of the middle child goes unnoticed, often leaving behind a frustrated young child.

To take care of this frustration, the middle child often makes many good friends his or her own age ... not too old and not too young. Since middle children do not have their parents all to themselves, they quickly learn to get their way by careful and skillful negotiations and compromise. Middle children are often very good at counseling others on how to get along in life.

Studies have also shown that middle children are very likely to be a faithful spouse. Because of their own family upbringing, middle children are very sensitive to correcting many of the problems that they experienced. In other words, middle children are loyal, eager to stay committed, attempting to make sure that their family feels included and wanted.

While there are certain inherent weaknesses of middle children, their strengths include being learned, unspoiled, realistic, loyal, trustworthy and willing to do things differently, knowing how to get along with others, as well as being good at mediation and peacemaking. And that pretty much describes my middle child Tommy.

However, while the book on birth order was very informative, it did not really answer Tommy's question. The simple answer is that I had not written about Tommy because, quite frankly, he was not the first or last to leave home, not the first to marry, or the first to present me with a grandchild. He is the middle child and second son, and this put him at a certain disadvantage in stimulating an article ... until now.

Personally I think it would be a good idea for all parents to learn something about birth order. While not a perfect science, birth order does seem to effect many of our traits, which in turn, effect our lives.

There seems to be a clear distinction between being the first, middle or last born, as well as being an only child. Perhaps, had I known about the implications of birth order when my children were young, I would have taken more pictures of Tommy. I certainly would have written a newspaper column about him sooner.

• • •

WHEN OUR CHILDREN BECOME ADULTS

Sitting in a large University of Georgia auditorium in Athens several years ago with family and friends to witness the graduation of my youngest child Catherine, I was filled with a sense of pride and love. My little girl had finally grown-up.

Becoming a grown-up was important to Catherine. I remember the many times, after reaching her 18th birthday, she pleaded with me or Julie to go somewhere or do something based on the argument, "You know I am a grown-up now." The law, which allowed her to vote and serve in the military, may have considered her a grown-up, however, I certainly did not.

Walking across the stage, shaking the Dean's hand and accepting her diploma, I thought that it was finally time for me to agree: my 22-year-old college graduate was finally a grown-up and had now reached adulthood. Or had she?

A recent study conducted by the University of Chicago, surveying 1400 American adults last year, reported that most believe adulthood does not begin until a person finishes school, gets a full-time job, gets married and starts raising a family.

Those surveyed were asked to break these criteria down by age and reported that the average age should be for: finishing school, 22.3; attaining full-time employment, 21.2; being able to support a family, 24.5; getting married, 25.6; and having children, 26.2.

The majority of those surveyed believed that adulthood begins at the age of 26. Catherine may have grown-up, but in the eyes of most Americans, she was not yet an adult.

Times sure have changed. In the 14th century, William Manchester pointed out in his book, A *World Lit Only by Fire*, girls married and gave birth as soon as they reached puberty, usually at the age of 13. Of course, in those days, few lived beyond the age of 30.

Even as recently as the 1950s, couples commonly married at the age of 18 with the blessing and acceptance of family and society.

Now, however, there exists what some experts are calling an "extended adolescence."

Society expects our young children to attend college, even pursue post-graduation education avenues such as medicine and law and encourages waiting to get married and having children. In short, Americans are supporting this extended adolescence process.

It appears that this extended adolescence may soon be extended ever further than it is today. Graduating college students are finding that there are few jobs available for them upon graduation.

Statistics reveal that only about 15% of these students will have jobs waiting for them, and with another 25% continuing their studies in professional schools, 60% of graduating college students have no long-term plans for employment or further education.

Without employment, many students are moving back home and becoming frustrated, anxious and confused. Adulthood for many of these young men and women seems far away.

While the national unemployment rate is approximately 6%, for those between the ages of 20 and 24, it is closer to 10%. How can our young men and women become adults, as defined by the recent survey, if they cannot find the means to become financially independent?

Our children are extending their adolescence by extending their education. For the first time in many years, applications to medical school are up as are applications to law and graduate schools.

Applications to "Teach for America," a program which recruits college graduates to teach in poor neighborhood public schools for two years, has tripled in the past few years. Even the Peace Corps has gained the attention of college students with more seeking to join this once extremely popular post-college learning opportunity.

But extending the time until our children become adults may not be such a bad thing: perhaps our children and society may even benefit from this delaying trip towards adulthood.

It was with all this in mind that I realized Catherine was, if not a real adult, certainly was now a grown-up. Although she extended her "adolescence" by continuing her studies in nursing school, I imagine she will fulfill the remaining criteria set forth by public opinion on becoming an adult.

In the meantime, while Catherine may not be an adult in the eyes of society, because she will be living away from home, voting, making day-to-day independent decisions and moving toward full employment, marriage and child rearing, she will nonetheless at least have joined the ranks of grown-ups.

Despite all this, however, until the day I die, she will always be my little girl.

• • •

IT'S ALL ABOUT GENES

I have always marveled at the uniqueness and variation of humans. Much like snowflakes, no two human beings, not even identical twins, are exactly alike. In an effort to explain our individual characteristics, experts have given us three basic explanations.

There are those who claim that it is our environment which dictates who we become and how we handle life's ups and downs. There are others who believe that it is basically our genetic coding that sets the stage for individual characteristics and traits.

Then there are those who insist that we are who we are because of both of these factors. I have always believed that this third explanation was the most reasonable and plausible to accept.

However, while environment most certainly plays a role in affecting and directing our personalized traits, it seems our genetic make-up often dominates who we are, how we act, what we feel and how we live our lives.

Using similar genetic testing principles and techniques as those used to isolate the genes responsible for a variety of illnesses, such as cystic fibrosis and breast cancer, geneticists have isolated a gene for anxiety, as well as one that is associated with the desire for excitement (the so-called bungee-jumping gene). These discoveries are only the tip of an enormously large iceberg.

Genetic scientists may someday announce the discovery of a gene or series of genes for temperament, courage, anger, desires, loquaciousness, passion, moodiness, happiness, and perhaps even sexual orientation, to name just a few.

A gene-based explanation for someone's personality is not too far off in the future. Each cell in the human body contains approximately 30,000 genes spaced along the 46 chromosomes which have already been isolated and identified. Only a fraction of these genes have so far been identified, but in the next several decades most will probably be discovered.

These genes, working in billions of combinations, are responsible for who we are to a larger degree than we had previously thought.

While it may take a few genes to stimulate an angry response in someone who has just been cut off in traffic, there are in those individuals with a slow or blunted response to anger, a set of more powerful and influential genes that overrides this impulse. The absence of such calming genes in some may help explain those whose fuse is quite short.

Personally, I am comforted by this evolving theory of a gene-based personality. It means we obtain our personality characteristics honestly. And although it by no means takes away responsibility for our actions, it does explain much of what and why we do specific things.

Although we develop from our genetic pool, our environmental factors also contribute to who we are and influence our behavior by episodically stimulating or suppressing our genetic composition. This would help explain why some children raised in a very negative environment turn out to be very special successful human beings, while even though raised in an extremely positive one, others turn out to be total failures.

Environment, however, does not seem to have any significant dominant or long-lasting effect on our personality. Who we are and who we become is to a very large degree dependent on the genes we possess or lack.

I probably lack the anxiety gene, which would explain why I am basically a non-worrier and an even-temperamental kind of guy. I certainly lack the bungee-jumping gene, for there is no way I would ever do such a thing, much less parachute from a plane, traverse a mountain, or drive a racing car.

I had always thought I was just a chicken. Now I know it really is not that at all. It is my genes that are saying "no way." That certainly sounds like a better explanation to me.

• • •

THE "BIG CHILL" WEEKEND

If you have never watched the *The Big Chill*, I suggest that you make renting this over 20-year-old movie a priority on your list of things to do, and treat yourself to what has become an American movie classic.

It is the story of eight former University of Michigan graduates, now in their 30s, brought together by the suicide of one of their college chums. It is set in Beaufort, South Carolina, at the home of one of the former students, now a wealthy shoe manufacturer. Each of them has an interesting story to tell since graduation.

Their weekend together speaks of unrealized dreams and shattered relationships, compromises that had to be made, and still promising hopes and expectations yet to come. It was a walk down memory lane back to the good old days of college.

Recently I walked down this same memory lane and had my own "Big Chill" experience. Fortunately, it did not take a death to get my former summer camp friends together once again.

While a few of us had maintained a relationship, the group as a whole had not been together for four decades. So we decided to get together to renew old friendships and catch up on how the past 40 years had treated us.

The Bradenton, Florida, home of a retired dentist and his artist wife, pleasantly located near the 13th hole of a beautifully manicured golf course and nestled between tall moss filled trees, became our movie set for revisiting the past, sharing the present, and looking to the future.

Unlike the movie characters, however, we were considerably older, and much more comfortable with ourselves. Our conversations seemed to focus more on sleep patterns, cholesterol and blood pressure levels, where and when we were to have our next meal and, of course, our children. Our future appeared clearer, perhaps because, in many ways, it had become our present.

Instead of focusing on what we wanted in the future (as did *The Big Chill* characters), our stories were filled with details of our pasts. We mostly talked about what we had wanted to accomplish in our lives and what we had actually achieved, as well as what we still hoped to find in the years yet available to us. We also talked about the many mistakes we had made along the way.

Although the characters in the movie were friends in college, they had grown apart and seemed uncomfortable with each other. A few of them had become successful in their fields, while several of them were still searching. Together they did not fully trust each other to understand and approve of who or what they had become.

Our "Big Chill" weekend was different. Each of us had the satisfaction of having our past neatly tucked away and we were comfortable with who we were, where we had been, and what we were doing.

We had completed the first journey of our lives and had fun talking about where we were going from here. Our defenses did not need to be guarded. We knew and accepted each other and could be who we were without concern of criticism.

We had known each other as teenagers, and little about any of us had seemed to change. We had formed a friendship many years ago at summer camp in the hills of North Carolina, and it had withstood the test of time and separation.

So we used our two days together to re-connect and share stories. We still liked each other and found comfort in each other's presence. There was no chill in our togetherness.

The Big Chill characters spent their time together evaluating their current life choices, talking about whether they were headed in the right direction in attaining their dreams. They were young and still could make major changes in their lives. Our group of eight spent our time reminiscing about our life's choices and whether the choices we made had fulfilled our expectations.

Our group had gathered together to take stock of our lives, to compare what we had done and to share our experiences with trusted old friends. It was a snapshot of the present now superimposed over a similar picture taken 40 years ago.

We also gathered together to talk about things to come, places to visit, books to read, art classes to attend and grandchildren to play with and hug.

Socrates once wrote, "The unexamined life is not worth living." As each of us travels life's path, I believe we should, on occasion, revisit the past and take stock of where we came from, where we are and where we still want to go.

We should do this in an environment away from the maddening turmoil of every day life, away from traps that keep us from a centering process, and we should do this in the company of old friends. This place should be able to allow spontaneity of talk and feelings and one that creates a suspension of time.

My weekend journey with friends of a former time helped enrich my journey through life. When I finally reach my destination, I will look back and know I traveled with hopes and dreams, with joy and love, and also with friends.

• • •

AS OLD AS YOU FEEL

There is an old saying that "you are only as old as you feel." Well, that is only partly true. You are also as old as you think you are.

I came to that conclusion, nine years ago, on my birthday as I walked along a sunny beach in Florida. My birthday usually finds me in a pensive, reflective and contemplative mood, so it was natural for me to begin thinking about the fact that at the age of 56, I was slowly, but surely, heading towards what many call old age.

But exactly how would I know when I had reached this golden milestone in life?

If I am truly as old as I feel, I thought, then on this particular day I felt 56-years-old. My muscles were increasingly stiff in the morning and my joints ached at night. My back was causing me considerable problems, and spicy foods were no longer agreeing with me. I awoke several times in the night, and tired easily by late afternoon, while frequently finding that I had little stamina for extended evening activities.

And just like my father in his mid 50s, I was noticing that ever-so-familiar male abdominal bulge, despite exercising and watching what I ate. In short, I felt 56-years-old.

Yet, despite feeling 56 physically, my brain kept telling me I was only 35, and this was causing problems for me. For example, thinking I was 35, I thought nothing about challenging a high school friend of my daughter, who was on the track team, to a 100-yard dash. Despite warnings from my daughter, since I had run this event in high school I believed I could at least hold my own and maybe even impress her. Embarrassment was more the result!

At about 80 yards into the race and with my opponent yards ahead of me, I tore my left hamstring muscles and spent weeks in rest and rehabilitation.

Another time, knowing I was in shape and thinking I was invincible, I thought nothing about running five miles on Saturday and three miles early Sunday morning followed by a competitive game of racquetball with a friend on Sunday afternoon.

Into the third game, my fatigued muscles took over causing me to fall and tear my Achilles tendon which resulted in surgery and six months of cast, crutches and rehabilitation.

There is more. Despite increasing back pain while jogging, I just could not accept the fact that my running days were coming to an end, until one day after a particularly long run, I could not get out of bed for three days. I was thinking 35, but I was feeling 56.

And so, on that birthday walk, I made a resolution. I would try very hard to let my body tell my brain what it can do rather than the other way around.

These past nine years I began doing what I have told so many of my patients to do. I listened to my body. Instead of jogging, I took up walking. Instead of racquetball, I began playing tennis because I found it easier on my muscle and joints. I gave up eating spicy foods and began going to bed earlier at night, while adding a 20-minute nap to my afternoon regimen.

These past few years have come and gone, and as I found myself walking down that same stretch of beach recently on my 65th birthday, I realized that this strategy had indeed worked. While I still thought younger than I felt, I felt much better thinking smart.

• • •

THE SORROW OF LOSING A PET

It has been said that the most difficult loss is the loss of one's child. While I am sure that is true, the question of which loss of life is the most painful to endure is really not a contest.

Many years ago, a patient of mine, whose husband of 52 years had recently died, exclaimed that her loss was the most painful process she had ever endured and that nothing could be quite as painful. The loss of someone you love cannot be measured in degrees of pain parameters. It is equally true even when that loss is a pet and not a person.

A few years ago Julie and I lost our 8-1/2-year-old dog, Sheba, in a tragic accident. We are still grieving. I was surprised at the intensity of our grief, but perhaps I should not be. Sheba, at times seemed human-like in understanding my moods and needs. Displaying unconditional love, she brought us immeasurable joy and happiness.

We missed her when we were away from home and often had trouble leaving her with others on our many trips out of town. Each time we left the house, Sheba had that look on her face that said, "Please take me with you." Seeing her run towards me when I returned home, tail wagging and head down eager to accept my affection, Sheba taught us the simple unconditional aspect of love. Her loss has created an emptiness in our life.

Seventy million Americans have household pets, with the majority considering their animal to be a member of the family. My three children were grown and living in other cities and Sheba was like having another child in the house. She joined Julie and me at dinner, took daily walks with us in the neighborhood and lay at the foot of our bed as we slept.

Word of Sheba's death seemed to travel almost as fast as when my parents died. Sheba may have only been a dog, yet her untimely death stimulated an amazing and unexpected amount of caring and support.

Julie and I were both surprised and overwhelmed by the outpouring of sympathy from colleagues and friends. We received dozens of condolence cards, emails and phone calls from friends around the country, as well as flowers and donations in Sheba's memory to the Nashville Humane Society.

As I soon discovered, there are an enormous number of pet lovers who understand the incredible effect that pets can have on us and how much love they can bring into our lives.

Even though we know that when we bring a pet into our life we are bringing into our hearts a life that more than likely will end long before our own. We accept this fact because we also know that the pleasure brought to us during the years our pets live is well worth the pain that follows when that life ends.

Statistically pets have been shown to bring incredible comfort to the elderly in nursing homes and senior housing. Pets can also bring comfort during times of grief and sadness.

The feeling of love that pets bring can stimulate even the most cynical and injured heart. Though not human, they bring out our own humanity in ways that other people often simply cannot.

Perhaps someday we will own another dog, although I seriously doubt that we will. Sheba was the most loving and smartest dog I ever owned. She could never be replaced. Dog and cat lovers know what I mean when I say that the relationship between human and animal transcends almost any other.

When I was alone with Sheba, I was not alone. I was with my best friend, my confidant and ally. She is missed in ways that remind me of others I have lost during my life.

The loss of a child has to be the most intensely painful, with the loss of a spouse, parent, family member or dear friend equally high on that list. However, the loss of a pet still ranks high enough to cause significant pain and anguish. That says something about the special relationship between humans and their pets.

• • •

THE GOOD OLD DAYS ARE NOW

I marvel at the ability of humans to properly function while being totally unaware of their surroundings. I am referring specifically to that car ride home, when suddenly you arrive and realize you don't remember the actual drive or any familiar landmarks passed. Despite the fact that your mind was obviously deep in thought and somewhere else, you were still able to send appropriate signals to arms, legs and eyes to allow safe passage through heavy traffic, changing lights, and stop signs.

Unfortunately, many of us too often go through life with much the same experience. We work and play, yet are really not aware of our surroundings or any real aspect of the experience itself. We do not savor the moment and, therefore, cannot truly bring awareness to an appropriate level.

In other words, we often go through life much like that car ride, suddenly finding that life is over and that we had not really been aware to enjoy the moments.

It is not that we have not been told to be more aware. Go to the self-help section of any bookstore, and the point of becoming more aware is made over and over. It is, however, not easy to train oneself to become aware. It is a feat that must be practiced repeatedly before it can become a daily part of life's routine.

Many years ago, having read a book entitled *Be Here Now, Now Be Here*, I realized that I needed help in learning how to live in the here and now. Too often I found I was aware of entering the hospital in the early morning and leaving later that night. I had acted robot-like during the in-between and, therefore, had lost an important part of my life.

Thus, I began training myself to become more aware. Each time I used my pocket watch to check time, or when I merely felt it nestled in my pocket while going about my daily routine, I used this symbolic event to cause me to stop and begin an awareness process.

This process included how I was feeling, what was happening, and in general, noticing the many wonderful things that were taking place around me.

Years later, I was able to put aside my watch as a triggering process and enter this awareness phase spontaneously each day.

Too many of us have difficulties living in the present. We glorify the past and look to the future to give us pleasure or peace.

Katherine Graham, at the end of her book, *A Personal History*, stated it well: "I am grateful to be able to go on working and to like my new life so well that I don't miss the old one. It is dangerous, when you are older, to start living in the past."

The good old days are now, not then. And Winston Churchill, reflecting as a youth on the subject of life after death, also stated it well. "People who think much of the next world rarely prosper in this." Living for the future robs one of the value and worth of the present.

I believe one should become more aware of each and every moment of our lives. We must awaken from our sleepwalking by sharpening our senses.

With only a little practice, we can visualize the many beautiful aspects of life around us; we can truly taste each bite of food, smell wonderful fragrances of nearby flowers. We can feel the wind in our faces, rain on our cheeks and snow on our tongues.

Our lives should not be a mindless, unaware drive home through heavy traffic. Heightened awareness has the potential to bring good mental health and help us through physical illness while enriching our lives.

• • •

LIFE'S BOOKENDS

"Birth is a beginning, death a destination and life is a journey." This opening line of a religious prayer for those mourning the death of a loved one has always interested and intrigued me. It seems to put into simplistic terms the essence of all our lives.

We are born, and then begin to travel along a journey towards our ultimate and final destination. The phrase, for me, emphasizes the journey, the crucial aspect of our lives, with birth and death placed conveniently as bookends of our journey through life.

Many of my friends and patients have told me of their intense fear of dying. Being a physician has given me a unique opportunity to witness this process of death and dying, and to discuss with many individuals the journey they have traveled as well as the process of dying.

Through this experience I have come to realize that many individuals begin to feel as if their journey is over once they have been told of a diagnosis such as cancer that more than likely will result in their demise.

I prefer to believe the journey does not end until the last breath is taken and the last beat of the heart has occurred.

The clock of all our lives is in never-ending fashion slowly ticking away the moments of our day-to-day existence. Those, however, who have been told of a serious illness or pending demise, hear this ticking much faster and more loudly than the rest of us.

Yet the turned-up volume and speed of ticking in our ears should not detract us from realizing that the journey still continues, still winds itself along the curves of our existence, however uncomfortable at times, toward that destination called death.

While I have never been favorably impressed with Timothy Leary, the man who urged a generation of Americans to turn on, tune in and drop out, I was impressed by his comment noted by the press several years ago. Leary, 74, the former Harvard psychologist who became a celebrity in the 1960s for praising the use of LSD, was told he had inoperable prostate cancer.

"How you die," he stated, "is the most important thing you ever do. It's the exit, the final scene of the glorious epic of your life. It's the third act and you know everything builds-up to the third act."

He further stated that he looked forward to the real challenge of ending his life with dignity. Leary, despite his years of drug usage, still seems to understand the Yogi Berra premise that "It ain't over 'til it's over."

The journey may change, but until life has ended, fulfillment, pleasure and joy can still find a place alongside the anxiety, apprehension and pain. It is precisely because of this belief that I have steadfastly been opposed to physician-assisted suicide.

It is also why I firmly believe our journey, despite its ups and downs and its eventual association with the aging process, is a truly wonderful trip.

I am forever reminded of a patient with far-advanced cancer of the breast whom I was caring for many years ago, while working at the City of Hope in California, who was receiving chemotherapy on a weekly basis. During one of our visits I inquired about how she was doing. Her tumor had spread to her lungs making it difficult for her to speak.

Words came slowly and with great effort, yet her response still rings in my memory. She uttered with a smile a single word "wonderful."

Somewhat taken aback, I remarked how interesting it was that such cheerfulness filled her at a time of such obvious illness. She replied, "The best thing that every happened to me, doctor, is the day I was told I had cancer." "How could that be?" I asked.

"Well, doctor, before I was diagnosed with cancer I never really saw the sunset, I was never really aware of the wonderful things that life has to offer. But since that day, knowing that each day was limited and therefore precious, I began to notice the sunset and the sunrise; I heard sounds I never heard before; I smelled fragrances, tasted foods and touched textures as never before; all at once I became alive and richness filled my everyday."

With eyes slightly moist I finished my exam. As I turned to leave she added, "Just think of it, doctor, you could start all that today without cancer."

Three weeks later she took her last breath and died quietly in her hospital bed. As I pulled the sheet over her placid face, I knew that I had been taught a great lesson — one I would not forget.

My patient embodied the concept of living the last portion of her life, the journey, with understanding, acceptance, dignity and, yes, even joy. She understood the true meaning of the prayer that begins "Birth is a beginning, death a destination and life is a journey."

・・・

LIVING TOO LONG

Being in my 60s, I am noticing that the topic of conversation among many of my friends of similar age eventually focuses on the subject of longevity. It seems everyone wants to live a long, meaningful, happy life with the operative word usually being long.

I often wonder, however, how long is long and is there such a thing as too long? Clearly, we all know how to define a life that ends too early, but have we individually or as a society addressed the other end of that continuum of the days of our lives?

A recent visit to my 100-year-old aunt stimulated my thinking on this question. The oldest of my late mother's sisters, my aunt and I have always been very close, and I am blessed that our relationship is filled with love and concern for each other.

Despite her age, my aunt has retained a sharp and clear mind with an intact short- and long-term memory. Our regular conversations remain as they have always been, enjoyable and enlightening.

However, during the past few years the aging process has clearly limited her activities and taken its toll. My aunt developed a serious eye disease and is now legally blind in both eyes.

Except for an evening meal downstairs, she is confined 24-hours-a-day to her small one bedroom apartment in a senior housing unit unable to read books, newspapers or watch television. The radio and telephone are her only regular means of communication with the outside world.

While she has three caring and nurturing grandchildren and ten great grandchildren who bring her considerable joy when she is occasionally with them, her only child, two husbands and most of her former family and friends are all dead.

I sat with her in her living room on my most recent visit and we talked about her feelings concerning life. "I have lived too long," she exclaimed, however admitted that she is resigned to the fact that she can do nothing about her deteriorating condition other than live out the remaining days of her life regardless of the limitations, restrictions, boredom and loneliness that characterizes each and every day.

Other than her loss of vision, however, she is physically and mentally healthy. A fact that does not bring her any joy.

I was depressed as I packed to return home following my all too brief two-day visit. As we stood in the doorway of her apartment, I took her into my arms, gently hugged her small frame, kissed her cheek and whispered "I love you" with moisture quickly filling the rim of my eyes. In words reminiscent of my childhood days, she responded, "I love you too, Frankie."

I wanted so desperately to change the fact that this very special, loving and caring woman was of the opinion that she had lived too long. Helpless, I turned and left her standing alone in that dark small space she calls home.

Unlike many elderly people, my aunt does not feel she is a burden to her family, nor is she depressed or in pain. Yet despite all this and because of everything else that has happened to this remarkable woman, she feels as if she has lived long enough. She has made peace with her God and is prepared for the end of her life. She is ready and eager to die.

As we reach our senior years, perhaps that is the only way for any of us to determine when enough is enough. Perhaps that is the only true measure of when life is too long.

• • •

SPIRITUALITY AND HEALTH

As a young medical student in the 1960s, I do not recall any of my teachers ever discussing the issue of spirituality and its effect on patient welfare. It seemed to me then and for several decades after my training that physicians tended to avoid the subject of religion and spirituality altogether.

In fact, there seemed to be an element of hostility when the medical profession was confronted with patients who depended as much or more on their belief system than on their own physician.

Fortunately, there were some physicians who understood the importance of spirituality in medical practice and had the strength of their convictions to openly state their opinion. In 1910, Dr. William Osler, a famous and highly respected physician stated that "The subject (spirituality) is of intense interest to me. I feel that our attitude as a profession should not be hostile." There were others who also felt this way, but they were clearly in the minority.

Sadly, it was not until the last few years that the issue of addressing spirituality in the practice of medicine reached academic medical centers where students of medicine are taken through the rigors of becoming a doctor.

A person's spiritual feelings can be separated from a person's religious background and training. There are many in our society, who, while professing little interest in organized religion, are nonetheless quite spiritual in their approach to handling many of life's ups and downs.

When serious illness strikes, there are few atheists in hospital beds and many who dig deep into their spiritual core to find inner peace and support.

The medical profession is slowly, but surely, embracing the concept that physicians need to be attentive to a patient's religious or spiritual needs, as well as learn how to intertwine these needs into the overall approach to medical treatment. Medical organizations and boards of accreditation now require that spiritual needs of patients be considered and openly addressed.

But now that the issue of spirituality is being discussed and attended to by the medical profession, is there any proof a patient's use of religion or spirituality improves outcome? The best answer to this question is we are not sure.

One reviewer noted that 75% of 325 studies indicated that religion improves health and well-being. *The Handbook of Religion and Health* published in 2001, reviewed 1200 articles with similar findings. The major problem with all these studies is most lack a proper scientific research approach and therefore cannot be accepted as evidence-based medicine by the medical profession.

While there are many intriguing studies on the effects of spirituality and religion on medical outcome, there are no definitive answers that meet the rigid criteria needed to convince scientists or skeptics. I have taken the position, however, that if a patient believes that their spiritual tools can help, then that is all the proof one needs.

If that "help" is one of bringing inner peace and strength as well as acceptance of one's illness, then I believe that is a positive result. A well-known writer on the subject once stated, "If you are a believer you don't need proof and if you're a skeptic you won't accept proof."

Spirituality and faith seems to work by giving the patient a sense of hope and control. Hope and control can reduce stress and create a sense of inner peace, as well as evoke beneficial changes in the body, such as, decreasing blood pressure, breathing and metabolism rates, and improving the body's immune response.

What we also know from large surveys is that 80% of Americans believe spiritual faith or prayer can help patients recover from illness or injury and more than 60% think that doctors should talk to their patients about faith and even pray with those who request it.

How then can doctors best address this controversial subject which lacks absolute scientific proof yet remains an important tool for patients to use in times of medical crisis? Guidelines to answer this question are emerging.

Physicians should take a spiritual history from adult patients in order to determine whether spiritual beliefs are used by the patient to cope with illness as well as to determine if these beliefs would in any way influence medical decisions. By obtaining this information, physicians will be able to provide support for religious beliefs when they do not conflict with necessary medical treatment.

I have noted that most of my patients have welcomed discussion of spiritual issues and that a dialogue on this subject enhances overall communication with my patient.

The medical profession has come a long way in being encouraged to discuss spirituality with patients since the day I entered medical training. We still, however, have a long way to go. Infusing spirituality into medical care may not be the only answer in obtaining a cure, it may, however, be part of the answer.

• • •

THE POWER OF TOUCH

During my third year in medical school, I was exposed to a teacher who, as a specialist in Internal Medicine, had earned the reputation as one of the finest diagnosticians Vanderbilt Medical School ever had on its faculty.

One of the most important lessons I learned from this doctor was the lesson of observation. He taught me that listening to my patients was only one way to hear them, and that patients would tell me more with their body language than they ever would with their words. How right he was!

Over the past 35 years I have continued to sharpen the skills of observation and improve my ability at reading the language of body and soul and as a result, I believe this ability has made a difference in the care I have been able to give to my patients.

Attempting to see past mere words spoken by my patients, I was often able to visualize physical and emotional pain that was so close to the surface. Sometimes it was the manner in which words were spoken, other times it was a faint hint of moisture in a patient's eyes or simply the manner in which a patient moved while speaking.

It was as a patient myself when one such observation occurred. A few years ago, following surgery for a torn Achilles tendon, I required six months of rehabilitative physical therapy which involved frequent sessions each week to regain my strength, range of motion and ability to walk unaided. During this time I observed an interesting phenomenon in myself, as well as other patients around me who had a variety of handicaps, and were having similar sessions with their physical therapists.

That phenomenon was one of dependence by the patient on the physical therapist and parental-like behavior of the physical therapist toward the patient. This resulted in an extremely caring, nurturing and even tender relationship.

Patients and therapists around me seemed especially friendly to one another. One could palpate the feeling of goodwill, friendship, caring and concern and one could also witness a genuine aura of warmth throughout this big room where a dozen or more patients were working with their therapists.

Witnessing this interesting relationship, I could understand the special relationships that developed between patients and therapists, as occurred in the movie *Regarding Henry*. Henry, having sustained a gunshot wound to the head and requiring specialized intense physical therapy to regain his ability to talk and walk, developed a warm and nurturing relationship with his therapist. Their relationship revealed a special depth of human need, support and comfort that continued even after Henry's hospitalization ended.

Although that movie was fiction, I am told that across this country, patients and their physical therapists do in fact develop similar relationships reflecting this special bond, often culminating in long-term friendships and occasionally even in marriage.

It seems to me that this observation is best understood and explained by the simple fact that the patient who is injured, handicapped and struggling to regain function and composure, becomes extremely dependent on his or her therapist to achieve this goal.

The therapist, in turn, feeling needed and respected on one hand, and feeling the vulnerability and helplessness of the patient on the other, is understandably drawn to a feeling of closeness and concern.

However, I think there is an additional explanation for this unique relationship between patient and physical therapist. Perhaps it's due to the fact that physical therapy is one of the few remaining aspects of medicine that includes the laying on of hands. The frequent touching that is involved with physical therapy certainly can be given credit in helping explain this unique relationship between patient and therapist.

Despite all the high technology that is available in medical care today, the laying on of hands, the touching of the patient is still crucial in the healing process. I am glad my professor in medical school emphasized keeping my eyes open to human behavior. I certainly would not have wanted to miss this one.

• • •

HOLDING ONTO HOPE

The ringing hospital phone startled me. As an intern I had spent many nights in the hospital lounge. On this particular night I had just fallen asleep, when a nurse, needing help with a very agitated, distraught and tearful patient, decided to call me for advice. After listening to the situation I decided to go to our patient's bedside and see if I could help.

Earlier that day, we had operated on this lovely and eloquent middle-aged woman to remove a suspicious tumor of the ovary, which was discovered during a routine gynecological exam. What we found surprised us all.

The tumor was malignant and had spread to many areas of her abdomen, including her liver. We did what we could, but each of us around the operating table that morning knew that our patient would more than likely die in the next year and there was little that we could do to change that.

It was now up to the patient's private physician to begin the process of explaining and informing both the anxious family in the waiting room and then, as soon as possible when she awoke, the patient.

After completing the surgery, my teacher (the patient's physician) asked me to follow him from the operating room to the waiting room. As we made our way down the hall the family quickly surrounded us, their faces revealing fatigue, anxiety and fear.

I watched with amazement and respect as my teacher took them to a quiet room and, with considerable sensitivity and careful attention to words and phrases, explained what was found, what could be done, and that despite the ominous findings there remained an element of hope.

As we left the room he turned to me and said "Always leave some hope in the room, it's sometimes the only medicine we have."

Later that same day, when the patient was awake and alert her nurse informed us that she was ready to be told what happened.

Standing next to the bed in the recovery room and listening to her physician explain, I was once again impressed.

Ever so slowly he gave details in such a way as to be understood easily, while explaining what he had found and what would be the next steps. Whenever possible, he reassured. Finally, he took her into his arms and told her how sorry he was that she had to go through this.

After we left her bedside he turned to me again and said "The only words that work here are I'm sorry. Don't try to say more."

Moments later, over a cup of coffee and in a somewhat pensive mood he continued to explain that he felt our job as doctors was to help our patients clearly and openly understand what was happening to them and with sensitivity help them through the inevitable stages of dying.

He emphasized that we had to understand the importance of these stages and know that patients needed to deal with each stage on their own time schedule and in their own way. Our job as physicians was to support them and be good listeners.

The hope he believed important to leave with his patient and her family that day, was not the hope of a cure. My teacher explained to me that the hope he wanted to leave with his patient was the hope of acceptance, control of pain and peace.

Each day alive is precious, he exclaimed. "I hope our patient can find peace and closure to her life. This is the hope I wished to leave her with."

That lesson helped me as I sat on the patient's bed that early morning, holding her hand and listening to her grief and disbelief pour forth. It was reassuring to me as a young physician to know that I did not need to say anything more. Just listening would work and that when it was time for me to say something I would know what to say. I learned much about medicine that day. I learned how a physician should handle the probability of death without overlooking the possibility of life.

Being a good physician is more than diagnosing the end of one's life, it is also helping patients with life until that life comes to an end.

• • •

HEALING WITH WORDS

The three most powerful words humans can say to one another are "I love you." These three simple words can transform a relationship from causal to intense, dramatically lift the spirit of those who hear them, and have the ability to heal both new and old wounds.

To say "I love you" brings to the recipient a sense of comfort, security, and peace, as well as, a feeling of being wanted and needed. Find three other words that can do all that!

"I love you" needs no qualifiers or adjectives. "I love you" stands alone, apart from all other words and phrases. Its strength lies in its simplicity and meaning.

To say "I love you" expresses a feeling so rich and profound that little else matters and all else is stripped away from the inner core of one's soul and being. If words can be perfect, then "I love you" are perfect words.

All too often we abuse these perfect words, from using them to try to achieve sexual favors to selling beer ("I love you, man"). Sometimes these words are used when we are not certain they express what we truly feel, making them meaningless, common, or mundane. But what's even more unfortunate is when these words aren't used at all.

Love should never be taken for granted. It must be nurtured and expressed in such a way that those we love are constantly reminded of our feelings of love for them. To show love and to speak love is at the core of a loving relationship and, as shown by a study of women with coronary heart disease, can also be at the center of improved health.

Swedish scientists, reporting in the *Journal of the American Medical Association*, noted that among a group of 292 female patients between the ages of 30 to 65, who were hospitalized for heart disease and then followed for approximately five years, that those women who experienced marital stress had a three times higher rate of recurring and worsening heart disease than those women who did not experience marriage difficulties.

Even when the scientists corrected their data for age, education, smoking, diabetes, estrogen status, blood pressure, cholesterol levels, and basic heart function testing, they still noted that women who complained of marital discord were more likely to have worsening heart disease over time. Interestingly, this same group of women was not adversely affected if they experienced stress at work. The problem, it seems, is at home.

Each woman studied answered a series of questions in order to evaluate the level of stress in their marriage and at work. The first of 17 questions relating to marriage was "Is the relationship with your spouse loving?" While other questions inquired about the level of friendliness, togetherness, trust, and sexuality, I consider this first question the most significant.

A marriage described as loving is one in which each partner feels loved. While feeling loved does not necessarily require being told of that love, it certainly can't hurt to be occasionally reminded.

The authors of this interesting and important study wrote "that marital stress worsens prognosis in women with coronary heart disease is consistent with previous findings that lack of perceived social support in women is associated with increased risk of first and recurrent acute myocardial infarctions (heart attacks), and that it is consistent with reports of an adverse effect on lipid levels and glucose metabolism in women." They even attempted to explain these findings as well as their own by speculating on the "potentially damaging effects of negative emotional states and/or stress on neuroendocrine and physiological regulatory mechanisms." (A medical way of saying stress can cause progression of disease and can kill.)

It seems that the stress of a bad marriage can also cause progression of coronary heart disease and can kill. Women who considered their marriage riddled with stress were more likely to suffer increasing coronary artery blockages, heart attacks, or death, than those women who considered their marriage a loving one.

This brings me back to where I began. The three most powerful and healing words that we can say are "I love you." Say it often and with conviction. Who knows? It may save a life.

• • •

HEROES IN MEDICINE

In a society that seems to concentrate on the flaws of individuals, it is becoming increasingly difficult to find a contemporary, workable definition of a hero. While Webster contains a list of attributes that make up its definition, I prefer to pick and choose from its list to define my heroes of medicine, with achievement, courage and sacrifice clearly my top choices.

There are the obvious heroes beginning with the Father of Medicine, Hippocrates, who, well before the common era, founded a tradition of medicine that emphasized clinical observation and ethics; the Greek philosopher, Galen, whose studies in physiology and anatomy around 170 A.D. remained widely influential until the late 16th century; William Harvey, the British physician of the 17th century, who accurately explained how blood circulated through the body; Edward Jenner, who in the 18th century found and administered the first effective vaccination against smallpox, a practice that has wiped out this dreaded disease; William Morton, who gave the first demonstration of ether as an effective anesthetic, thereby ushering in the field of anesthesiology.

There are other heroes: Rudolf Virchow, the German pathologist, who around the middle of the 19th century published the book Cellular Pathology in which he discussed his discovery that disease occurs at a cellular level; Louis Pasteur, who described how germs can cause illness and disease, and then who later used his findings to develop pasteurization, a process that significantly improved health of the industrial age population; Joseph Lister, Ignatz Semmelweis and Oliver Wendell Holmes, who described how deadly infections could be prevented by antiseptic techniques.

There was William Roentgen, who at the end of the 19th century discovered x-rays, thereby creating an entire new field of medicine; the German chemist, Felix Hoffman, who introduced the incredible drug aspirin to the world; Karl Landsteiner, the Australian pathologist who discovered major blood groups and worked out a system that resulted in safe life-saving blood transfusions; Paul Ehrlich, in the early 20th century, who found a cure for the dreaded syphilis, thereby establishing contemporary chemotherapy; Frederick Banting, the Canadian surgeon who in the 1920s isolated insulin, a landmark discovery for the treatment of diabetes; Alexander Fleming, the British bacteriologist, who in 1928 discovered penicillin; George Papanicolaou, who developed the now famous life-saving Pap smear to detect early signs of cervical cancer; Charles Drew, the American surgeon who in 1940 described how blood plasma could be stored; William Kolff, the Dutch doctor who developed the first artificial kidney dialysis machine.

The list continues: the Americans, James Watson and Francis Crick, who won the Nobel Prize in Medicine in the early 1950s for their discovery of the structure of DNA, the molecule that carries our genetic coding; United States pathologist, Gregory Pinkus, who reported on the first successful studies of the birth control pill; the American Robert Gallo and the French Luc Montagnier, who each in the middle of the 1980s found the genetic sequence of the AIDS virus; and the United States geneticist, W. French Anderson, who performed the first gene therapy on a 4-year-old girl to cure her diseased immune system.

There are many other obvious heroes of medicine: Sigmund Freud, the father of psychiatry; Masters and Johnson, who introduced science and objectivity to the field of human sexuality; Christiaan Barnard, the South African surgeon who performed the first heart transplant; and Jonas Salk, the founder of the polio vaccine; William Halstead, the Johns Hopkins gifted surgeon; Sir William Osler, the incredible observant clinician; Edward Quilligan, a gifted teacher, practitioner and creator of modern obstetrics; Benjamin Spock, the visionary pediatrician; Michael DeBakey and Norman Shumway, talented and innovative cardiac surgeons; Edward Steptoe, the first to achieve a successful in vitro gestation; and Mildred Stallman, the visionary Mother of Contemporary Neonatology. I could go on and on.

Then there are the not so obvious or famous heroes of medicine. They are the dedicated men and women, who, at often a huge financial cost and commitment to long and arduous hours of study, entered the field of medicine to become the everyday workers, spreading understanding, compassion and health to the world. You may not know them all, but you know a few. They are the real heroes in my opinion.

They "practice" medicine because they are perpetual students, always learning better ways to administer their healing techniques. They are the teachers of the next generation of doctors, ever so carefully nurturing their entrance into the honored profession of medicine. They are the researchers constantly evaluating new ideas, technologies and treatments to improve the health of their patients. They are the men and women who sit at the bedside after many sleepless hours, listening, prodding — while holding your hand — in an effort to heal and bring comfort.

Let society search for flaws in humans. They will find many. I prefer searching for those who achieve, have courage, and sacrifice. These are my heroes.

• • •

PRACTICING MEDICINE

I have practiced medicine for 41 years and during this time I have often been asked why doctors "practice" medicine? While there are several ways to define the word practice, a common understanding of what practice means is "to do repeatedly in order to learn or become proficient." But the question always remains the same, "Shouldn't we already be proficient when we become doctors and no longer need to practice?"

The truth is that doctors practice all the time. We are in a constant mode of learning to do it better, to become more proficient. We can never learn it all. In that sense, the practice of medicine is quite humbling. In our ever changing world of medical advances and new technology, a truly good doctor is always practicing.

We practice by reading medical journals each month, attending lectures and postgraduate courses each year to learn what is new and effective, undergoing re-certification exams to prove to others that we still have what it takes to be proficient and, most importantly, by looking at each patient as a challenge that needs careful scrutiny and attention so as to wind up with a good result. I was reminded of this when I was on call at the hospital not too long ago.

Melinda was 34-years-old and 26 weeks pregnant when we met. She was in our care because she had insulin dependent diabetes, a blood clotting disorder and, tragically, because she had lost all of her six pregnancies, three by miscarriage and three stillborn babies. The three babies that died in Melinda's uterus prior to birth were at 30, 28 and 26 weeks gestation (a normal pregnancy is usually around 40 weeks). What was particularly worrisome was the fact that no one knew for sure why her babies died inside her uterus at those times or what could be done to avoid this current pregnancy ending the same way.

During her last pregnancy we had attempted tight control of her diabetes and testing her baby twice a week to ascertain its oxygen reserves. Despite all this, Melinda came to us a few days after all tests looked reassuring with a baby that had died in her uterus at 26 weeks.

So, here she was once again pregnant at 26 weeks gestation with no answers from our medical team of high-risk doctors how to assure this pregnancy would have a different outcome. We felt we had given her the best available medical care possible during her last pregnancy and didn't know what more we could do.

I explained this to Melinda and her family. But I also told her that since we did not know what was causing her babies to die, we would try something different. We admitted her to our hospital and tested her baby every day, in every way we could. We took nothing for granted. Melinda accepted our plan as we began a rigorous course of testing her fetus in multiple ways each day for its ability to remain alive inside her uterus.

As we made our rounds each day, we carefully reviewed each test that was performed for any changes or signs of problems. As long as everything remained the same, we were reassured. While Melinda's child was not growing as fast as expected, her diabetes was in good control, her blood was properly thinned and daily heart rate monitoring and ultrasound testing of her unborn child did not reveal any problems.

Then quite suddenly after three weeks of hospitalization and at 29 weeks gestation, my resident called me. "Dr. Boehm, I need you to look at Melinda's tests." I quickly went to Melinda's room and looked at a fetal heart rate pattern that looked troubling and an ultrasound exam of a baby that was not moving, a potentially ominous finding. A mere 24 hours earlier, Melinda's baby appeared healthy, but now things were very different. A quick decision to perform a Cesarean Section was made and within minutes we delivered Chelcie, a two pound six ounce baby girl who seemed dazed but healthy.

Later, while talking to a very happy mother and family, I still could not understand what had happened. What I do know, however, is that all of us at the hospital that day were thankful for the delivery of a live and healthy baby. I also knew that we had all been reminded of the important fact that practicing medicine was a continuous learning process, and that while we do not always understand the complexity of the human body, we can respect and learn from that complexity. That's why I love the practice of medicine.

. . .

DOCTORS: TOO FEW OR TOO MANY?

It is not a question often asked by the American media, yet it is an increasingly important one to address. Are there enough doctors in America to take care of us now and in the future?

Currently, there are approximately 800,000 actively practicing physicians in the United States, a number considered by many experts to be too few to adequately take care of the current population, and especially in the very near future when we will have close to 80 million baby boomers (born between 1946 and 1964) reaching senior citizen status.

The number of graduating medical students in this country has remained constant since the 1980s despite the fact that the US population has since grown by 50 million to its current 300 million. The Council on Graduate Medical Education has gone on record to recommend training 3,000 more doctors each year, and the Council's Chairman, Carl Getto has stated, "Almost everyone agrees we need more physicians. The debate is over how many."

For the past 25 years, the American Medical Association had claimed that we have too many doctors, and in 1994 stated that by 2000 there would be a surplus of 165,000 doctors in America. They were wrong, and we are now suffering the results of their predictions.

To their credit, the AMA has stepped back from its earlier position and now states that we will need more physicians in the future to take care of an ever increasing aging population. Even the Association of American Medical Colleges has dropped its prediction of a growing surplus of doctors and has stated, "It now appears that those predictions may be in error." The organization now recommends a 15% increase in the number of graduating medical students. It seems that we now all agree. We need more doctors.

There are currently 126 medical schools in the country

graduating approximately 17,000 students each year. Add to this group a large number of foreign medical students entering postgraduate training and we wind up with about 25,000 new doctors entering the practice of medicine each year. The problem is that although today these new doctors equal the number of doctors retiring, within approximately 10 years the number of baby boomer doctors will begin retiring in larger numbers creating a significant shortage of needed physicians. Add to this the fact that doctors are working shorter hours than in the past, are reluctant to go into specialties in which malpractice is a concern, and reluctant to go to remote parts of America, and you can understand why so many experts are concerned that we are heading for a significant physician shortage in this country.

To be fair, there are dissenting voices to the call for more doctors. Some experts believe it is foolish to think that more doctors will care for under served populations or will go into needed specialties. Many experts also claim that physicians create their own demand and are concerned that more doctors will only drive up the cost of medical care by ordering more tests and performing more procedures without improving the health of America.

Don Detmer, co-chairman of an Institute of Medicine committee, has claimed that, "If we produce an abundance of doctors, there's little incentive for the system to become more efficient." That opinion is countered by the argument that it is also foolish to limit the number of physicians in this country as a means to control health care costs. Preventive health measures and illness is what drives health care costs today, not doctors.

So what can be done to assure Americans that there will be an adequate number of doctors to care for us in the years ahead? To begin with, we can increase the number of students in existing medical schools all across America. We did that once before in the 1970s when, because of a perceived need for more doctors, each medical school class was doubled. My class at Vanderbilt in 1961 contained 52 students. Within 10 years it had grown to 104, a number that persists today. There are thousands of qualified premedical students turned away from medical schools each year. Most, if not all, of the medical schools could begin accepting more students without lowering standards of a first class education.

In addition, we could also increase the number of medical schools. Florida State became the first new medical school in this country since 1982 and will graduate its first class this spring. Other schools in California, Arizona, Nevada and Florida are also interested in opening new schools. It is time we encouraged them to move ahead.

These measures will require government help and will take time and money. However, it is critical that we act now. Too much is at stake to do otherwise.

• • •

THE PRICE OF BEING A DOCTOR

During teaching rounds with medical students a few weeks ago, one of our patients asked the students why they had chosen to become doctors. Before anyone could answer, the patient's mother spoke up. "The reason is to make money." Over the years I have heard this many times and was not surprised with her response. The problem, however, is that she was wrong.

Money is actually one of the last reasons young men and women choose medicine as their career. How do I know this? First of all, money was never a consideration when I chose to become a doctor, and over the past 40 years I have heard this from thousands of medical students and doctors I have taught and worked with.

The main reason given for choosing to become a doctor is a love of science and a desire to help others. Doctors, as a general rule, are not interested in the business world but are motivated by a thirst for knowledge of how the human body works and how to maintain and improve the health of patients. It is not that we do not care about making a nice financial living, it is that we do not spend much time thinking about it as we go about our daily chores. Surveys have shown that many doctors have no problem in being placed on a salary or even being paid by the hour.

Keep in mind that the average debt of graduating medical students in this country is $120,000. Most new doctors take on even more debt as they continue their medical education as residents and fellows. It takes about 10 years to fully train a doctor in the United States and, therefore, it is not unusual for doctors leaving training and entering private practice to owe over $200,000.

Once in private practice, young doctors find that expenses to run an office and to pay medical malpractice fees seriously reduce their annual income. In addition, much of that annual income is dependant on what specialty the doctor practices. Doctors who practice primary care medicine such as Family Practice, Pediatrics or Internal Medicine make considerably less money than those physicians practicing a surgical sub-specialty or Cardiology and Gastroenterology.

The average net income for a primary care doctor in 2003 was $146,000 while Surgeons who specialize in areas such as orthopedics had an average net income of $271,000. Payment to doctors reward physicians who become Surgeons, Cardiologists or Gastroenterologists who perform procedures or tests, in contrast to doctors who spend their time evaluating and diagnosing without being able to perform procedures. As a result, the median income of a doctor who is a General Practitioner in 2004 was $120,000; a Pediatrician, $145,000; a Family Physician, $146,000; an Internist, $150,000; an Ob/Gyn, $215,000; a general Surgeon $230,000 and a Cardiologist $250,000.

It should be noted that these figures are averages and many doctors make considerably less as well as more. These numbers illustrate that while doctors overall make a very comfortable living, considering the long educational and training process which results in huge debts, coupled with incredible responsibilities of the job, as well as long working hours and the need for continuing education and recertification on a regular basis, the amount of remuneration is not outrageous as it seems in some arenas such as the corporate world.

It was recently reported that the average income of physicians decreased by 7% from 1995 to 2003 after adjusting for inflation. (This is in contrast to lawyers whose income during this time rose 7%.) Currently Medicare plans to cut physician payments by 5.1% next year and as a result many doctors in primary care specialties are wondering if they can maintain their practices.

It is a good thing that young men and women interested in becoming doctors do not put money as their top priority for making their choice.

• • •

NOTHING HAS CHANGED: BUSINESS AS USUAL

In 1999, the prestigious Institute of Medicine published a report entitled To Err is Human, which claimed that up to 98,000 deaths occur each year in United States hospitals due to errors made by health care providers. This astonishing report pressured the health care industry to make changes that would correct the problem of errors made in the care of hospitalized patients. Now, seven years later we learn that the number of deaths that occur each year in American hospitals have actually increased, perhaps even doubled! It appears we are back to business as usual. What is going on here?

It is not that the health care industry has not tried to correct the problem of medical errors; rather it has not been focused on the real issues causing medical errors. This assessment comes from two distinguished experts on the subject of medical errors writing in two prestigious medical journals.

In The New England Journal of Medicine, George J. Annas writes that he believes the law should recognize patient safety as an inherent right. He believes it is the responsibility and duty of all hospitals to make sure that this right is protected and hospital responsibility can become a major motivator for developing systems in hospitals to reduce medical errors. This, Annas states, is contrary to the popular premise that it is lack of tort reform to reduce liability that is the real barrier to putting into place hospital safety programs. Annas goes on to say that "Hospitals that do not take specific actions to improve safety should be viewed as negligent and be subject to malpractice lawsuits when a violation of the right to safety results in injury."

Annas also believes that all hospitals in America should put into place a system of reporting all errors, as well as what he calls near misses for quality control, which is to "make sure patients are told when their injuries were caused by errors." He does not believe that universal reporting and being open and honest with patients will drive up malpractice claims since no study has yet shown that reporting medical errors has increased medical malpractice rates.

Vanderbilt is one of the few hospitals in this country that has made a patient's right of safety a top priority. We are working with system management groups in an attempt to change the culture of doing business with our patients. Initiating a computerized mechanism to place medical orders in a patient's chart (which has resulted in a significant reduction in medication errors), and hiring consultants from the highly effective safety conscious airline industry to work among doctors and nurses to put into place processes that lead to reductions in communication and system errors, are two examples of how Vanderbilt has taken seriously the right of a patient to safety.

Annas's bottom line is that with a national adoption of a patient's right to safety, hospitals will be more likely to take measures to meet a goal of safety since failure to do so would result in increased liability to the hospital.

Dr. Louis Weinstein, writing in The American Journal of Obstetrics and Gynecology, also addresses the issue of preventing medical errors. He claims that, "The emphasis of most physicians and medical professional societies has been on seeking tort reform with the imposition of non-economic damage caps and contingency fee limits." He believes the medical community needs to spend more effort on preventing errors than attempting to reduce liability for medical errors. He has a point.

Medical errors that lead to patient harm are most often system errors and, therefore, with determination and a will to change, amenable to repair. Weinstein believes that tort reform does not address medical errors that are preventable, and also believes we should remove the privilege of non-disclosure of peer review systems in hospitals so as to regain public trust.

Without an open dialogue with our patients, as well as implementation of many other processes to effect patient safety, we are doing nothing to put into place a system that will result in a reduction of hospital errors (while increasing lack of trust in the medical profession). The recommendations by these two experts on the subject may be controversial but at least they are addressing the untenable situation of an increasing rather than decreasing number of medical errors that lead to patient death. We need to pay more attention to what they say.

• • •

GENETICS AND PAIN

Over the years I have witnessed thousands of women give birth and I have found that people have many different reactions to pain, and that pain is an extremely complex process.

For a long time I have believed that a person's reaction to pain would someday be proven to be heavily influenced by genetic factors, and that we will learn that there are genes which express our ability to handle pain. The identification of these genes will help us understand why some patients have an extremely low threshold for pain while others a very high one. Now there is information that gives support to this belief.

Reports of a small number of people throughout the world who do not feel any pain, give convincing proof that genes play a major role in the perception of pain. A condition called congenital insensitivity to pain with anhidrosis (CIPA) is a rare genetic disorder inherited from both parents that makes an individual unable to feel pain or adapt to extreme external temperatures. CIPA disrupts the development of nerve fibers which transmit sensations of pain, heat and cold to the brain. It renders the body incapable of a critically important protective alarm system.

While you may think that the inability to feel pain is a good thing, let me tell you, it is not. Individuals who are unable to feel any pain are in extreme danger of serious harm. Imagine if your appendix ruptured and you could not feel pain and therefore did not seek medical attention. What would happen if you fell and broke a bone or touched a hot stove and could not react with a quick response of moving your hand? Children afflicted with CIPA have to be continuously watched at play and adults have to carefully monitor their bodies for unfelt injuries.

Much of human behavior is on a continuum with extremes on either side of average. Sexual preference, intelligence, athletic ability and temperament are a few examples. The fact that a condition exists which renders an individual incapable of feeling pain caused by a genetic disorder, explains why there are some individuals, at the other end of the spectrum, who are very sensitive and incapable of handling even the smallest amount of pain. The majority of us fall somewhere in the middle of this wide continuum of pain perception.

Because of this genetic connection to pain we should be more tolerant of those who seem to be the most intolerant of handling pain. They are most likely not weaklings or complainers, but rather genetically endowed with an extremely efficient nerve response system, the very opposite of those inflicted with CIPA.

The medical profession should teach its practitioners that pain is not only subjectively perceived and expressed; it is also affected by a more objective modality of genetic expression. In other words, a patient who states that her headache or labor pain is a ten out of ten should be treated as if that pain is truly severe. It is also important, when confronting a patient who claims their pain to be minimum, to still consider more serious pathology if other clinical factors suggest it.

All this is not to suggest that pain is only expressed through genetic factors. Consider the impact of prayer on pain, or that of the placebo effect. Recently it was reported that patients with severe migraine headaches responded positively to acupuncture when it was properly performed, as well as when it was not. In an article of the Journal of the American Medical Association, it was reported that 51% of patients had significant reduction of the pain caused by migraine headaches when they underwent properly administered acupuncture, while 53% of similar patients also noted reduction of pain even when the acupuncture needles were placed at non-acupuncture points.

Clearly, pain is a complicated process and one with which the medical profession constantly struggles. We have improved our evaluation of pain and are making headway in treating it as well. It is still important, however, for both doctor and patient to understand that the management of pain remains one of the most significant ingredients of good medical care.

• • •

EMERGENCY ROOM MEDICINE

In 1969 while working in southern California, I needed to be able to fly my family home to Nashville for visits. Because I did not have the money to pay for our flight, I did what many young doctors often did in those days, I signed up to work two 24 hour shifts in a nearby hospital's emergency room. In those days, you see, there were no doctors who specialized in Emergency Medicine so emergency room positions were filled with doctors needing or wanting to make some extra money. How times have changed!

The first residency programs to train young doctors to become specialists in Emergency Medicine began in the mid 1970s and have grown ever since. Today the field of Emergency Medicine has become an equal to other specialties such as Surgery, Medicine, Pediatrics, Obstetrics and Gynecology.

Emergency rooms are now staffed by men and women who are highly trained to care for the critically ill and to handle the most complicated of emergencies. American medicine is the better for this relatively new specialty. Despite all this expertise and professionalism, however, Emergency Medicine Departments in this country are in trouble.

In many ways emergency rooms can be compared to canaries in a coal mine. A canary that dies in a mine is an early warning to working miners that the air is dangerous and that they should immediately exit. Emergency rooms are dangerously troubled today and represent an early warning sign that indicates our health care system is dying, and that we must exit our current way of administering medical care and begin making significant changes.

The reason is clear. Patients are coming to emergency rooms for minor medical conditions as well as serious problems. Because so many Americans do not have a primary doctor, they must rely on emergency rooms for routine care. This has created a serious problem for doctors and nurses as they attempt to decide who needs urgent treatment opposed to those who could wait.

Due to the large number of Americans without health insurance and huge cost increases in medical care, emergency rooms are seriously over crowded and close to the breaking point. The number of patients seeking care in emergency rooms has increased from 90 million in 1993 to 114 million in 2003. It is even higher today. In addition, 423 Emergency Departments throughout this country have closed.

All this has resulted each year in over half a million ambulances being diverted from emergency rooms that are full to others further away. It is estimated that many people have died as a result in a delay in treatment as well as not receiving treatment in the chaotic environment of an overcrowded ER.

We are witnessing a large influx of patients who are seeking routine medical care and are uninsured and cannot find a doctor to take care of them. They have no place to turn for help and so they come to the ER. By law, hospitals cannot turn away any patient seeking care regardless of whether they can pay or not.

Considering all this, one wonders how we are going to be able to deal with a major disaster such as a mass casualty or influenza epidemic. How will we be able to get the kind of emergency care we need when the time arrives?

It is time to respond to the canary's demise in our emergency rooms. We need to put together a system that will allow all citizens to have health care insurance and thus be able to obtain primary care outside the ER. We need to increase the number of doctors graduating from medical schools and make it attractive financially for more to chose primary care specialties as well as to practice in poor neighborhoods.

We also need to stop diverting real emergencies and begin diverting those who are seeking non-emergency care to neighborhood clinics staffed by round-the-clock doctors or nurse practitioners. All this will require a will to act as well as money. Yet we must act if we are to save our emergency departments.

• • •

OBESITY AND HEALTH CARE COSTS

Recently I viewed a video of a Cesarean Section performed on a woman who weighed 650 pounds! (Her baby weighed a normal 7 pounds). While I have had patients whose weight was in the 400 pound range, the video was alarming as well as troubling. Unfortunately, Americans are getting larger and larger each decade. It has been reported that the incidence of obesity in America has increased dramatically over the past 20 years, and that one out of every three women in this country is now considered obese.

Keep in mind that there is a difference between being overweight and obese. The World Health Organization defines normal weight as a body mass index (BMI) of 18.5-24.9; overweight 25-29.9; and obesity, greater than 30. To calculate your BMI, which uses height in inches and weight in pounds to determine results, just go to Google.com and type in BMI and use their calculator.

The woman, in the video, undergoing a Cesarean Section had a BMI significantly over 40, a figure considered in the extreme or morbid range and was at an alarming increased risk for serious medical complications. Obesity in women of childbearing ages is related to an increase in miscarriages, stillborns, premature births, fetal spina bifida, overly large babies, diabetes mellitus, hypertension and toxemia of pregnancy. In addition, the Cesarean delivery rate increases as a woman's BMI increases; reaching almost 50% in women whose BMI is 35-40. Postoperative complications are also higher in obese women and include a higher incidence of excessive blood loss, longer operative time and an increase of wound infections. Obesity is not just a problem for pregnant women.

Obesity for the general population is associated with an increase in death rates and in one study, an estimated 112,000 individuals die annually of obesity associated causes. Besides an increased incidence of deaths, obesity has been associated with an increase in type 2 diabetes, hypertension, heart disease, gallbladder disease, osteoarthritis and a number of cancers, including breast, uterine and colon. In other words, obesity kills as well as causes serious illness for a large population of Americans.

However, in addition to an increase in death and disease, obesity is costing Americans a huge amount of money spent on obesity related medical problems. In order to take care of obese patients, hospitals have to build special beds, chairs, toilets and operating beds, simply to be able to admit extremely obese patients and perform surgical procedures in a safe manner. The added cost to care for hospitalized obese patients is a problem for hospitals throughout America.

Clearly, this increase in obesity is part of the reason the average cost for a family health insurance policy has now reached almost $11,000 a year, according to a survey conducted by the Kaiser Family Foundation. Growth in medical insurance costs is now higher than growth of work wages as well as inflation. We cannot continue to add higher costs to what individuals and families must pay each year for health care insurance without continuing to add to the already swollen number of medically uninsured Americans.

The Kaiser survey noted that only 60% of employers offered health care coverage, down from 69% just five years ago. Most of the reduction comes from small companies, which cannot afford these kinds of costs for their employees. Many large companies with over 200 employees, who do offer health care insurance and who pay an average of 74% of an employee's plan, are attempting to reduce their overall costs by giving incentives to reduce high risk behavior affecting general health, such as smoking, lack of exercise and over eating. Employees who lose weight and thereby avoid certain obesity related illnesses save money for the employer. All this, however, will not be enough.

Obese Americans need to wake up and understand that they are killing themselves. The medical community can only do so much. This is not so much about being somewhat overweight but rather about being in the obese category as determined by one's BMI. We need to find a way to help the one-third of our population who are obese, tackle their weight problems. It will not be easy, but it has to be done.

• • •

CONFLICT OF INTEREST IN MEDICINE

I have a question for you to ponder this morning. What significant ethical issue does the medical profession and political community have in common? If your answer is conflict of interest, you are correct. It turns out that conflict of interest for physicians is a real problem in this country, similar to that which exists for politicians.

Approximately 2500 years ago Hippocrates wrote his famous oath for physicians to take before embarking on a medical career. That oath has been modified over the years, most recently by a group of doctors in the United States and Europe who produced a new oath called "A Physician Charter." This new Charter was written in an attempt to address issues which did not exist in ancient days, such as doctors being tempted by pharmaceutical and medical device companies to accept gifts and other inducements. The new Charter encourages doctors to avoid falling prey to the problem of conflict of interest by including a pledge to maintain trust.

In a landmark article the Journal of the American Medical Association (JAMA) defined conflict of interest. "Conflict of Interest occurs when physicians have motives or are in situations for which reasonable observers could conclude that the moral requirements of the physician's roles are or will be compromised." Financial conflict of interest occurs when a doctor uses personal financial gain to make decisions in patient care rather than what is best for patients.

In the JAMA article eleven influential doctors were critical of gifts, money and educational courses that the pharmaceutical and medical device companies routinely give doctors, claiming that these activities present negative conditions for patient care and that they should be banned altogether. Clearly, this is an important article and one that has already produced much discussion in the medical profession. But really how big is this problem?

In terms of money, it is huge. The pharmaceutical and medical device companies spend approximately $18 billion each year marketing their products to doctors. The goal for these companies is to entice doctors to use their products. In addition, the industry sponsors over 300,000 educational events each year for doctors, also in an attempt to induce doctors to use their drugs or medical devices.

This enticement includes, but is not limited to: gifts, meals, payment to attend conferences or lectures, travel payment to meetings, payment to be a part of a speaker's bureau, giving doctors free medical samples to give patients, consulting payments, ghostwriting services and grants for research studies.

While many medical professional organizations have provided guidelines as to how to handle this largesse by pharmaceutical and medical device companies, the authors of the JAMA article believe they are inadequate and do not work. These authors state that "The profession itself must exert much tighter control over the relationships between manufacturers and physicians."

Studies have shown that even small and or modest gifts to doctors influences a doctor's prescribing behavior, and that these gifts create an environment in which physicians will request certain drugs be added to a hospital formulary, or that doctors increase writing prescriptions of drugs (that may be more expensive and no more effective than other medication) manufactured by the company that gives the gift.

The authors of this important article further state that "Medical Schools and teaching hospitals throughout this country should be the first to establish a ban on all gifts and perks offered by the industry," and add that eventually all doctors need to address this issue and also establish a comprehensive ban. While it is true that many industry sponsored educational sessions for doctors are helpful, it is critical that grants given to support educational venues do not play any role in the content or participants of the course. Even with that stipulation, it is well-known that the pharmaceutical and medical device industry have influences on what is taught at many medical educational events for doctors.

The pharmaceutical industry employs approximately 88,000 sales representatives to visit doctor offices all across this country in an attempt to educate and influence prescribing practices. These "detail" men and women also hand out close to $11 billion worth of free drug samples. Patients who are begun on these "free samples" eventually run out and then need a prescription to continue remaining on the medication. The JAMA article recommends this practice be replaced with a voucher system that would place distance between the doctor and the pharmaceutical industry, something that Vanderbilt started several years ago and works very well.

I believe it is time for the medical profession to tighten guidelines on conflict of interest. Medical schools will need to monitor adherence to restrictions and guidelines and be prepared to enforce them. Eliminating all gifts from the pharmaceutical and medical device industry as well as assuring that grants and consulting funds are transparent and subject to peer review would be a good start. Patients need to know that when we take care of them, no conflict of interest exists. That certainly is a noble and worthwhile goal.

• • •

THANK YOU OR BRIBE?

I was delighted to learn recently that Stanford University Medical Center in California has bitten the bullet and adopted a policy that will prohibit its doctors from accepting even small gifts, such as coffee mugs and writing pens, from representatives of pharmaceutical companies. The policy goes even further in its restrictions and, make no mistake about it, this new and innovative policy will cost the medical center a lot of money. What Stanford Medical Center has done, however, is the right thing to do.

The Dean of the Medical School reported that the new policy would cost the Medical Center millions of dollars each year. Lost revenue will occur in part because the policy will not allow the pharmaceutical and medical technology industry to sponsor meals, to run medical lectures and seminars and will disallow doctors from accepting free drug samples as well as from ghostwriting medical articles that are published in medical journals. In addition, pharmaceutical representatives will be barred from contact with doctors in areas of patient care, and any physician who has responsibility in purchasing medical equipment will be excluded if they have any financial relationship with companies involved in contract bidding.

Each year the pharmaceutical industry spends $18 billion marketing to doctors to prescribe their drugs, and it works. Doctors who attend lectures when free meals are given, who are taken on educational trips and who are given even small and inexpensive gifts, are more likely to prescribe the company's medication or request that certain medical devices be purchased by the hospital. Often these medications and medical devices are expensive and not necessarily more effective than other brands and devices. In the short and long run, patients wind up paying a bigger price when doctors are influenced, for whatever reason, by the pharmaceutical and medical device industry.

It has been estimated that there are approximately 300,000 educational events sponsored by these industries each year in an attempt to induce doctors to use their drug or medical device. In addition, the pharmaceutical industry employs 88,000 men and women who are called "reps" and whose job it is to visit doctors in the hospital or in private offices to educate doctors on their product and urge them to consider prescribing their medication. Stanford's policy will stop that.

It is interesting to note that Yale University Medical Center and the University of Pennsylvania Medical Center have also adopted a similar policy. Other hospitals and teaching centers, including Vanderbilt, are considering such policies and I believe that more medical centers will adopt the policy of separating doctors from the seductive influences of the medical industry. During a time when the public is concerned about product and device safety as well as the rising cost of drugs and medical care, it is imperative that the medical profession remove any appearance of industry influence on the practice of medicine.

This new policy will not prohibit the pharmaceutical and medical device companies from awarding grants to medical centers for educational events. Strict guidelines already exist that prevents medical industries from influencing speakers or topics chosen for educational programs and each speaker must acknowledge any conflict of interest in writing and at the beginning of each talk if conflict exists. What Stanford's policy will do, however, is to prevent undue influence on doctors, young and old, from using drugs and devices that are not necessarily better and may actually be more expensive. It will also help build trust between patient and doctor.

It is time for all private practice offices and medical centers to adopt the policy that Stanford Medical Center just approved. It is the right thing to do.

• • •

PASSAGE OF TIME

As a young man I remember my father complaining to me about how fast time was passing. Being at the same stage of life as when he spoke these words to me, I can now truly understand what he was talking about. Time is passing faster than I can ever remember.

As a child I felt as if time stood still. School hours dragged on forever and summer vacation always seemed so far away. As an adolescent, each milestone of aging seemed to take forever to arrive, while college and medical school days seemed more like decades than merely four years each.

Time seemed to accelerate somewhat in my thirties and forties, yet I was not aware of feeling any motion as time moved forward. Suddenly, in my fifties, I felt a stir. Where had the time gone? How was it that my children were now fully grown and no longer living in my home? How did it happen that I was spending more time talking to my friends about health issues than about almost anything else?

Now that I am in my mid-sixties, time is moving even faster, causing occasional dizziness. Time feels much like a rewinding tape, beginning ever so slowly but gaining speed at it nears the end. When I wrote 2006 on my first check this year, it looked strange to me. Where has the time gone?

As I notice this acceleration of time, I try more than ever to enjoy and savor each moment of each day. Unfortunately, despite my attempts to become more aware of my days in hopes of slowing time, I do not believe I have been successful. And so I have come to realize that while I cannot slow time, I can at least live well as it rushes onward. After all is said and done, it is not how we start in life; it is how we end that really matters most.

With close to 80 million baby boomers (those born between 1946 and 1964) reaching these fast fleeting years, I believe this issue of ending well will become an important theme in our society. But what does ending well really mean?

It has been said that our days are like scrolls and that we should write on them only what we want remembered. As we age, it becomes imperative that we live our lives in such a manner that those we leave behind someday will remember us as kind, compassionate, honest, ethical and loving. Getting older also means getting smarter. As we age, we can avoid the many mistakes of our youth. We can do what is right and what will be remembered as noble and pure.

We can also take stock of our lives and begin planning to do the things we have always wanted to do: the trips we have not taken, the hobby or activity we have always wanted to participate in, the quality time we have wanted to spend with children, grandchildren or friends are just a few examples. There is much more for each of us to consider as we plan to end well.

We can set aside a special time each week to turn inward and reflect on the uniqueness of each day and the grandeur of our surroundings. The cathedral that God has given us needs our attention. A walk or hike in parks and meadows, fishing in a nearby pond, watching the sun rise and set, a sunset spin on a glass-like surfaced lake, or attending a place of worship on the Sabbath are just a few examples of how we can live and end well.

Most importantly, we need to take time to focus on those we love and to make sure that they know we love them. Love, after all, is the most important ingredient of living well. If there is love in our lives, each and every day will be enriched. If we enhance our days with awareness, fulfillment, integrity and love, then when the passage of our time comes to an end, those who know and love us will know we have ended well and that our time on earth was spent wisely.

• • •

ABOUT THE AUTHOR

FRANK BOEHM, M.D. is Professor of Obstetrics and Gynecology, former director of maternal/fetal medicine at Vanderbilt University Medical School in Nashville, Tennessee, and former chairman of the Vanderbilt University Medical Center Ethics Committee. He is a graduate of Vanderbilt Medical School and the Yale-New Haven Hospital Internship and Residency Program. His specialty is Perinatology (high risk pregnancy) and is recognized worldwide in the field of fetal monitoring.

In August 1997 *Good Housekeeping* listed him as being among one of the nation's best doctors for women in the field of Perinatology. Dr. Boehm was named in *The Best Doctors in America*, from 1992-2005, a referral guide of the nation's finest physicians based on peer nominations and recommendations.

In 2000 Vanderbilt University School of Medicine's faculty presented Dr. Boehm with the Award for Excellence in Clinical Teaching. In 2004 they also honored him with the establishment of the annual Frank H. Boehm Award for Excellence in Teaching for contributions to continuing medical education, of which he was the first recipient.

In 2004 he was also honored by the Vanderbilt University School of Medicine Department of OB/GYN with the establishment of the annual Frank H. Boehm Award for Excellence and Compassion in Perinatal Care.

Dr. Boehm's author credits include more than 200 scientific publications. He is the co-editor of *Assessment of Care of the Fetus*, a textbook in the specialty of maternal/fetal medicine, and serves as a reviewer of major scientific publications in his field.

Dr. Boehm has spoken on his specialty at conferences in the United States, Canada, Mexico, Europe and the Middle East. He is a member of the Vanderbilt Chapter of Alpha Omega Alpha, was awarded the Mead Johnson Award for Graduate Teaching, and in

1980 named Man of the Year by CABLE, an organization of Nashville business and professional women.

In 1992 he recognized the importance of helping patients understand the workings of the medical profession and the professionals in it. This led him to pen a column in the Nashville *TENNESSEAN* called "Healing Words" which he continues to write monthly.

Dr. Boehm's first book, *Doctors Cry, Too; Essays from the Heart of a Physician*, published by Hay House, is available at your local bookstore or online at www.DoctorsCryToo.com.

He and his wife Julie reside in Nashville and Boca Raton, Florida. He has three children, Todd, Tommy and Catherine, and four grandchildren, Riley, Adam, Marly and Seth.

Doctors Cry, Too: Essays from the Heart of a Physician

Doctors Cry, Too is a collection of essays from the heart of a physician which deals with issues surrounding health care and doctors. These essays portray a medical profession that is sensitive, emotional, spiritual, and compassionate. They include special moments in the life of Dr. Frank Boehm, such as a son and daughter going off to college, coping with the personal grief of losing loved ones, the birth of a granddaughter, and the healing that comes from joy. The essays also address his point of view on such subjects as strength and courage, faith, happiness, depression, forgiveness, death and dying, friendship, the heartbreak of infertility, parenting, and medical expectations.

It is the author's hope that *Doctors Cry, Too* will help the reader understand that physicians are subject to the same stresses and pressures of life, struggling with many of the same difficult and perplexing issues as everyone else, and that by gaining insight into the heart of one physician, the reader will gain insight into the heart of many physicians.

"Dr. Boehm has used a lifetime of experience in medicine to create a prescription for life we can all use. I cried, too." —**Art Ulene, M.D.**, author

"... Boehm's stories are filled with examples of what can happen when compassion is a part of the process. ... this book should be read by every present and future doctor and every patient." —**Bernie Siegel,** author of *Love, Medicine & Miracles and Prescriptions for Living*

"For many years I have known Dr. Frank Boehm as a great physician. *Doctors Cry, Too* proves with warmth and wisdom that he can also heal with his words." —**Crystal Gayle,** singer

"A loving and lovely book. It will remind patients to see their doctors as human beings and remind doctors of their obligation to be human beings first." —**Rabbi Harold Kushner**, author of *When Bad Things Happen To Good People*

Available at your local bookstore or our web site: www.DoctorsCryToo.com.